REMEDIAL MASSAGE THERAPY

REMEDIAL MASSAGE THERAPY

Eddie Caldwell

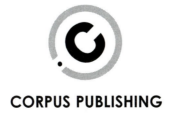

CORPUS PUBLISHING

First published in collaboration with
The Northern Institute of Massage in 2001 by
Corpus Publishing Limited
9 Roman Way, Fishbourne, Chichester, PO19 3QN

Disclaimer

This publication is intended as an informational guide. The techniques described are a supplement and not a substitute for professional tuition. Whilst the information herein is supplied in good faith, no responsibility is taken by either the publisher or the author for any damage, injury or loss, however caused, which may arise from the use of the information provided.

British Library Cataloguing in Publication Data
A CIP record for this book is available from the British Library
ISBN 1 903333 02 4

Acknowledgements
I feel a deep sense of gratitude to all the tutors (and guest lecturers) over the years from whom it was my privilege to learn about the art and science of massage.

I acknowledge my indebtedness to members of the Northern Institute staff and to students at all levels who have always taught me something or, at least, made me learn.

Mention, too, must be made of the rewarding relationships shared with so many patients, especially the 'pivotal' ones recorded anonymously in this book. They taught me more about the human body and its responses than anyone else.

"The sum is greater than the parts...."

Photography Gordon Crossley and Keith Allison
Anatomical Drawings Michael Courtnage
Text Design Tracey Shooter
Cover Design Sara Howell

Printed and bound in Great Britain by Bell & Bain Ltd., Glasgow
Distributed throughout the world by Human Kinetics – www.humankinetics.com – or:

USA
P O Box 5076, Champaign, IL 61825-5076, T: 1-800-747-4457, F: 217-351-1549

Canada
475 Devonshire Road, Unit 100, Windsor, ON N8Y 2L5, T: 1-800-465-7301, F: 519-971-9797

Australia
P O Box 80, Torrens Park, S. Australia 5062, T: (08) 8277-1555, F: (08) 8277-1566

UK and Europe
Units C2-C3 Wira Business Park, West Park Ring Road, Leeds, LS16 6EB, UK
T: +44 (0) 113 278 1708. F: +44 (0) 113 278 1709

New Zealand
P O Box 105-231, Auckland Central, T: (09) 523-3462, F: (09) 523-5462

Dedication

Marie, Katie, Chris, Rachel and David

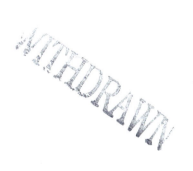

Contents

Foreword

I have probably known Eddie Caldwell for about twenty years. I certainly knew of him for more than ten years before that. He was a well-known professional wrestler and I played professional football. We both used to enjoy running and roadwork.

We shared many tales of how we both acquired a host of aches and pains and common injuries. I first met him personally when I was a young journalist – and later editor of the Bury Messenger in Lancashire.

By this time he was a qualified remedial massage therapist and he wrote a regular weekly advice column for my paper, providing a wealth of news, tips and information for thousands of sports men and women at the start of the running boom in the early 1980's. These articles became the foundation upon which we, with his wife Marie, co-authored 'Running for Fun', a book about running and running injuries.

I used to tell friends and colleagues that Eddie was the 'man with the magic hands'. It came as no surprise when he became massage therapist to England teams and attended at many prestigious international sporting events in this country and abroad.

His successful sports injury forums, mainly for runners, at which he used to graphically explain how injuries occurred and then demonstrate how to treat the injuries or prevent their re-occurrence are well remembered in the North West and North Wales.

A sought after remedial therapist, he always seemed to achieve the impossible and somehow repaired my torn or aching muscles in record time and allowed me to continue and enjoy playing football (at least on a friendly basis) and to be able to compete in charity marathons for many years afterwards.

He progressed from private practice into teaching massage techniques to aspiring therapists and some six years ago became the Principal of the Northern Institute of Massage, an institution with a worldwide reputation for the excellence of its tuition programme.

I feel honoured to have been asked to write this foreword for his book and I remain confident that the book will have a tremendous impact in the field of massage for many years to come. The book should be compulsory reading for anyone involved in the massage profession and will be an essential aid to massage students and newly qualified massage therapists.

Don Hale, *Editor of the Matlock Mercury*
'What the Papers Say' Journalist of the Year 2001
The Observer's 'Man of the Year' 2001

Introduction

The real value of the effects of remedial massage became apparent to me, not from what I read in books or what I was told by tutors, but from what my patients reported to me after their treatments. Upon completion of my training in remedial massage, I returned to my work in Special Needs with Manchester Education Committee and I had no intention of becoming a practitioner and, later, a teacher of massage.

I used my newly acquired skills to treat family and close friends, particularly members of the family and friends who were involved in various sports. I quickly became sought after to give what now might be described as post-event massage. Friends booked in for treatments after hard training weekends or just arrived back from competing in a marathon. They found that the aches and pains would be taken out of their legs or the discomfort eased from their necks, backs and shoulders.

The truth about the efficacy of the treatments slowly edged into my consciousness. The gratitude and praise, the talk of 'gifted' or 'miraculous' hands was being directed at my massage treatments and it took some time for me to realise just what my patients were saying. I only then became convinced that massage was a good form of treatment and I became more enthusiastic about developing a massage practice.

That year and against much well-meant advice, I resigned from my work after a career of some twenty years, took a mortgage on a bigger house and opened my first clinic in a converted garage. Not such a good idea, perhaps, with a wife and four children of school age. However, my patients had 'told' me that massage was an excellent treatment and that I would be kept busy enough to earn a living and meet my financial obligations.

It was at this time that I began to consider the merits of massage rather than just my ability to perform the various applications of massage. I realised that I had been most fortunate to have learned my skills at the best possible training school. Not only had my tutors taught me the art and science of massage, about anatomy and physiology but also about handling and managing people for their greater good and benefit. Traditions had been passed down to me via countless teachers and tutors and what I was passing on to my patients was the result of many years of experience, tradition and skill. Many hundreds of years, perhaps thousands.....

The more treatments I performed the more I wanted to find out about how massage worked, why it is so effective and why my patients responded so favourably and enthusiastically. I enrolled on more and more courses. I found out about manipulative therapy, the use of electrical therapy, the lymphatic system and how to treat it, the value of exercise linked to massage and many more aspects of massage. I know a few of the answers; many I do not know. One problem is how can you test the value of massage scientifically? Researchers have tried to do this in the past and the Northern Institute has embarked upon a research programme into the benefits of massage treatments in collaboration with the University of Central Lancashire and Professor Len Goldstone of The University of South Bank in London. Perhaps more answers will emerge as a result.

After establishing myself successfully in practice I was asked to teach massage and, later on, I became the Principal of the Northern Institute of Massage. Since it was founded in 1924, there have only been three Principals of the Institute. This is probably a very big factor in the ability of the 'Northern' to teach remedial massage in its purest form, via tutors and Principals who have striven hard to keep their standards as high as possible. This book is an extension of the tradition of passing on the information and the expertise to those who wish to learn. I pass on a lot of what I have learned from my teachers who passed on to me what they had learned from their teachers.

Eddie Caldwell
Principal, Northern Institute of Massage

Chapter 1
History of Massage

Massage – the Earliest Medicine

Massage is probably the earliest form of medicine and has been described as 'instinctive' medicine by both Woodward (1967) and Salvo (1999). It is ingrained in humans to rub the part that hurts, for example, after a fall. This technique has been with humans throughout the centuries. It is a natural response to rub our aches and pains whether or not we are familiar with the medical knowledge behind these actions (Salvo, 1999). Goldstone (1999) quoted Harris and McPartland (1996) who stated that the roots of manual medicine weave an arabesque back to pre-history. Massage or 'touch therapy', is described by Field (1999) as one of the oldest forms of treatment in the world.

The very derivation of the word massage is obscure and it is attributed by various sources to the Greeks, the Arabs and the French or least to the influence of French translations of ancient writings.

Tomb paintings, ancient carvings, manuscripts surviving for thousands of years and fossilised remains of massage oil vessels are testimony to the origins and development of massage through the ages. Salvo (1999) referred to European cave paintings depicting the use of therapeutic touch dating back to 15000 BC.

Hippocrates (460 – 375 BC), the 'Father of Medicine' preached the benefits of massage in his teachings… "hard rubbing binds, much rubbing causes parts to waste and moderate rubbing makes them grow." He also wrote that: "rubbing can bind a joint that is too loose and loosen a joint that is too rigid." An early indication of the therapeutic application of massage in which Hippocrates may well be referring to crossfibre friction to injured ligaments and the breaking down of adhesions around an injured joint. The Roman physician, Celsus, wrote that chronic pains in the head are relieved by massaging the head.

Galen, a Greek physician (I used to refer to Galen as 'Roman' until corrected with some vehemence by Alexander Adamidis, a colleague and massage therapist of Athens) worked in Rome as personal physician to the Roman Emperor Marcus Aurelius. He wrote many treatise about medicine, discovered arteries, helped establish a scientific application of massage and urged its use in the treatment of injuries and in the preparation of gladiators for combat in the arena. This latter application of massage finds a modern parallel in the pre-event aspect of sports massage.

Survival of writings about massage are scarce. Galen (131 – 202 AD), Avicenna (980 – 1037 AD), de Chauline (1300 – 1368) and Pare (1510 – 1590) also described the use of friction massage and its use in the treatment of stiff and injured joints.

A significant contribution to therapeutic and remedial massage was that of Ling (1776 – 1839) who is often referred to as the 'father' of modern massage. A Swedish professor of gymnastics and fencing, Peter Henry Ling established his school of massage in Stockholm where he taught a combination of massage and movements to promote general relaxation, improve circulation, relieve muscle tension and improve range of movement. The term 'Swedish Massage' is still used to denote the therapeutic application of massage.

To Metzger (1838 – 1909) and his students is generally attributed the classification of the principal massage techniques probably from French translations of Chinese books about massage – effleurage, petrissage, tapotement and friction. Kellgren, at the end of the nineteenth century added vibration to this list. Metzger was a physician and his teachings were more readily accepted than those of Ling who was not a 'mainstream' medical man. Goldstone (2000), in lecture, speculated upon the relative orthodoxy of Metzger and the acceptance of his methods by the medical 'establishment' because he was one of them, a doctor whereas Ling was a professor of Nordic Literature.

These early modern teachers were influenced by Hoffman (1660 – 1742) and his 'manuelle medizen'. He started the development not only of massage techniques but also manipulative techniques which developed into the osteopathic and chiropractic methods and including manual lymphatic drainage developed by Vodder some seventy years ago.

From about 1880, massage became very much a part of orthodox or mainstream medical treatment and was practiced by doctors and then by nurses. Prominent hospitals, for example, St. Thomas' Hospital, St Georges', Guys' and the Royal National Orthopaedic Hospitals had Massage Departments.

Nurses provided massage treatment under the direction of doctors and the Massage Sister was a familiar figure in hospitals. The private nursing services of major hospitals offered not only nurses but qualified massage therapists in the home.

As late as 1926, Goodall-Copestake wrote in the fourth edition of her book, *"The Theory and Practice of Massage"* that the science and practice of massage is in common use in almost every country.

Her dedication in the book is one from a grateful daughter in the memory of a physician – a faithful servant of God – a devoted student of his works and she acknowledged illustrations in her book from, *"Outlines of Massage"* by Goodall-Copestake. He was no doubt the physician father and one of the doctors who practised massage in the treatment of his patients.

After a period of much interest in and use of massage treatments in America, Europe and the UK during the latter half of the nineteenth century and into the twentieth century, there was a decline in the popularity and use of massage around the time of World War Two.

Salvo linked this to the development of pharmaceutical medicine and Goldstone (1999) with the growing influence of schools of physiotherapy, the profession of which has its origins in the Society of Trained Masseuses. The growth and professionalisation of physiotherapy and the introduction of electrical treatments saw massage gradually discarded. Jackson (1993) commented that it was very sad that the physiotherapy profession continues to exclude massage from its practice.

Woodward (1967) attributes the decline of massage in physiotherapy to its labour-intensive nature compared with electrical treatments. Woodward also pointed out that there remained in the UK, a hard core of massage therapists who believed in their work and who developed their practice of massage to a very fine art, achieving remarkable remedial results where other treatments did not perform so well. These unsung and sometimes unappreciated practitioners carried the standard through the years until the gradual swing back in the last twenty-five years. As well as the disappearance of massage from the schools of physiotherapy, Goldstone commented on the disappearance of the once common private schools of massage from the major cities of England.

Massage in its various forms and under a variety of names, for example remedial massage, neuromuscular massage, connective tissue massage, deep lymphatic treatments, sports massage among others, is often portrayed as 'alternative', 'complementary' and even a 'new' therapy. Goldstone (1999 and 2000) indicated that massage is not new or alternative; its long history is firmly within mainstream medical practice and was performed by doctors and by nurses under the direction and supervision of doctors. Goldstone's perceptive contributions to medical journals have suggested that massage is moving back into the mainstream of medicine via nurses and their growing use of massage and allied therapies in their work.

Massage has risen in popularity in the United States in recent years (Salvo, 1999). A detailed history and survey of the subject would take years and occupy a much larger volume than this. What has been shown in these few pages is a mere glimpse of the history and development of our therapy.

Chapter 2
Massage – Theory and Practice

What is Massage?

Massage has been described in various books and journals as the systematic and scientific manipulation of the soft tissues of the body. Many of the writers agreed further that massage is both an art and a science. To help towards a definition of massage the following references and quotations may be useful.

Goldstone (1999) quoted the definition by the American physician, Douglas Graham (1884):

"Massage.... is a term to signify a group of procedures which are generally done with the hands such as friction, kneading, manipulations, rubbing and percussion of the external tissues of the body in a variety of ways, either with a curative, palliative or hygienic object in view."

Massage is, stated Despard (1916), the scientific manual application of certain movements to the human body by which morbid conditions of the tissues are relieved.

Salvo began her book with the following statement: *"Massage is multi-dimensional – it is simultaneously an art and a science."*

The explicit connection between massage and hands is noted again by Tod (1951), who stated that massage, essentially performed by the hands, is a scientific manipulation of the soft tissues of the body. Tod described the movements or strokes of massage as the 'manipulations' of massage. This was echoed by Greenman (1989) who said that massage (manual medicine) is the therapeutic application of the hands in patient care.

Tappan (1988) referred to massage as the systematic and scientific manipulation of the soft tissues of the body and, though massage can be applied by electrical and non-electrical equipment, the techniques are primarily applied by the hands.

However, four different kinds of massage are listed by Menon and Asokananda (1999) in a description of massage techniques practiced in Kerala in India including Chavutti Thirummal or massage by feet for maximum pressure and effect. Other areas of Asia (notable among these are the techniques of Traditional Thai Massage) also have their own massage forms and techniques in which feet are used as the primary provider rather than hands.

More concisely, Rosser (1996) spoke of massage as the manipulation of body tissues to produce therapeutic effects. Whilst Field (1999) put an emphasis on the qualification and experience of the massage therapist by use of the word 'trained' in stating that massage is the manipulation of soft tissue by trained therapists for therapeutic purposes. Tucker (1969), whilst in no way devaluing the skill of the therapist, outlined massage treatments to be self-administered by the patient at home in cases of injury, rheumatism and osteoarthritis.

Types and Varieties of Massage

1. Remedial (Swedish) Massage.
2. Manipulative Therapy.
3. Lymphatic Drainage (Vodder).
4. Deep Lymphatic Treatments (Halliday).
5. Neuromuscular Massage.
6. Myofascial and Trigger Point Release Therapy.
7. Soft Tissue Release (Sanderson).
8. Traditional Thai Massage.
9. Indian Foot Massage.
10. Indian Head Massage.
11. Sports Massage.
12. Aromatherapy Massage.
13. Reflexology.
14. Rolfing.
15. Hellerwork.
16. Reiki.

17. Trager.
18. Touch for Health.
19. Shiatsu.
20. Muscle Energy Techniques.
21. Acupressure.
22. Ayurvedic Massage.
23. Bowen Technique.
24. Weir-Mitchell Treatment.

Massage Techniques

Effleurage

Perhaps the best known and most used of all massage techniques is effleurage, the stroking or gliding movement of massage. The word is derived from the French word effleurer which means, *'to flow or glide'* or *'skim the surface'*.

Effleurage is the massage stroke of initial contact with the patient and, as such, it is most important that effleurage is performed with great skill.

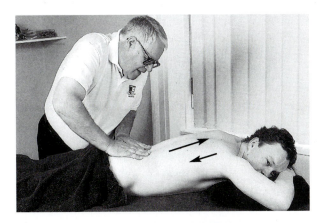

◀ *Figure 1*
Effleurage – the start position for back massage.

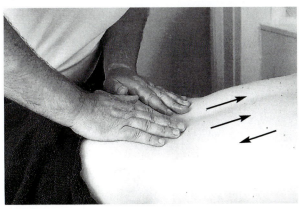

The patient's perception and reaction to this first contact with the therapist is one that cannot be repeated. The therapist will pass messages through his hands to the patient as the treatment starts. Touch pulls together the physical and the psychological and is so important in the therapeutic relationship (Mitchell and McCormack, 1998). Good technique is a necessity and poor effleurage technique will probably mean that the patient does not relax and will not be able to obtain benefit from the massage techniques that follow on from effleurage.

Effleurage and, indeed the other strokes of massage, stated Harper (1999) is not just rubbing the body. Each stroke has a specific action on the relevant tissue and this should be understood and appreciated by the practitioners whilst practised to perfection in order to achieve a good result.

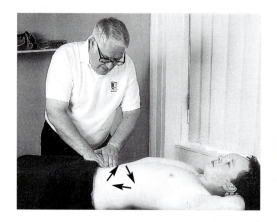
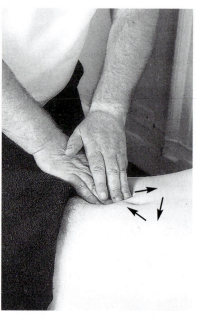

▲ ▶ *Figure 2*
Circular abdominal effleurage using
the whole palmar of both hands.

Effleurage is usually performed with the whole palmar surface of one or both hands. Where the area being treated is quite small, then the pads of the palmar surfaces of the fingers or thumbs may be used. The tips of the fingers are not used in effleurage. The technique may be used either in a superficial manner or much deeper according to the pressure applied by the therapist during the stroke.

Effleurage is mostly directed towards the heart, for example up the legs, up the back, down the neck. The pressure of the stroke should be applied in this one direction, the same direction as venous flow. Halliday (unpublished 2000) asked if this was a rigidly applied concept and should the directions of flow of the superficial and deep lymphatic vessels, which she stated do not always coincide with venous flow also be taken into account in the performance of remedial massage treatments.

The therapist should be relaxed and his hands must mould to the contours of the part of the body being massaged. The movement of effleurage must be rhythmic, smooth and unbroken and performed in a comforting manner and slowly if a relaxation is required or firmly and more briskly if a stimulating effect is required. Whatever the speed or pressure being applied by the therapist, a smooth and even rhythm is essential and jerky or uneven movements must be avoided.

As each effleurage movement is completed, the hands are returned to the starting point by lightly skimming them back over the skin with no pressure being applied. Thus the contact between the therapist's hands and the patient's body is never broken.

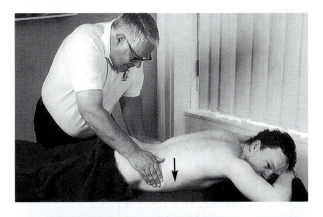

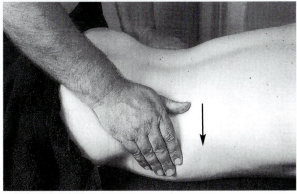

◄ Figure 3
'Lateralising' effleurage over the back.

Lifting the hands clear of the patient's body whilst returning to the starting point serves to disrupt the smooth rhythm of the treatment and the patient will not be able to attain the same level of relaxation. Do not remove the hands from the patient between strokes, but repeat the strokes successively with the pressure applied in the direction of the heart and the pressure taken off when gliding the hands back in the return movement.

By following this procedure it should be possible for the therapist to change, at the appropriate moment, from effleurage to the next technique in the sequence without breaking the rhythm or causing any discomfort to the patient.

When using effleurage to a large area of a body, especially if the person receiving the massage treatment is quite big, the therapist should not be static, i.e. should not stand in one place with feet firmly rooted to the floor. This will not only destroy rhythm, smoothness and pressure but will contribute to injury to the practitioner as he over stretches and strains his own body. I remind our students at the Northern Institute that Professor Ling was a professor of fencing and that he probably used his feet and body to excellent effect when massaging large bodies and/or large areas of a body. A little appropriate re-positioning of the therapist's feet will help keep the massage rhythmical, smooth and with the intended pressure from start to finish of the stroke.

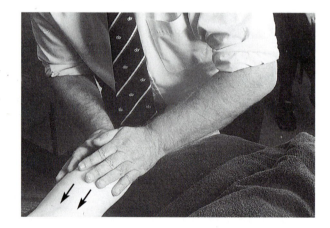

▶ *Figure 4*
Effleurage of the lower leg.

To the uninitiated observer, the effleurage movement appears to be a very simple movement to learn. However, as suggested previously, it requires a great deal of practise to perfect it. Too much or too little pressure is applied; the movements lack rhythm and smoothness; the hands lose contact with the patient; the therapist is not relaxed and his hands and fingers are not able to mould to the contours of the patient's body. A lot of practise is required and, for example, a tutor can tell within seconds of observing, the difference in technique between a student who does very little practise between practical classes and a student who practises on several people each week. It takes many months, even years of steady practise to perfect the art of effleurage.

Benefits of Effleurage

1. Helps relax the patient; has a sedative effect on the
    nervous or irritated patient.
2. Can help relieve tension headaches when applied to forehead and neck.
3. Soothes tired muscles.
4. Brisk effleurage, however, is stimulating and will increase blood flow.
5. Increases/stimulates lymphatic drainage.
6. Light centrifugal (i.e. from within outwards) can benefit
    some painful nervous conditions.
7. Assists venous circulation.
8. Prepares tissues for other, perhaps deeper treatments.
9. Soothes and 'normalises' after deeper treatment.
10. Has a stretching effect on muscles.
11. Many patients report it helps them to sleep after periods
    of unsettled sleep patterns.

The last point is a recurring item in discussion with patients after treatment. Many patients suffering chronic conditions, for example, shoulder injury or low back pain tell me that after the first treatment they experienced the best night's sleep they had experienced for a long time. Whenever a patient tells me this I feel like standing up and cheering. Invariably, that patient recovers well. The restoration of consistent sleeping patterns is one of the principal factors in healing.

Contra-indications to Effleurage

1. No massage should be applied to an area of the body where there
    is a skin infection or open sores or wounds.
2. Effleurage should not be used over varicose veins because of the danger
    of causing inflammation of the vein or perhaps even the formation of a
    thrombus. However, for the patient with varicose veins in the lower leg,
    massage of the upper leg would be beneficial in aiding general circulation
    of the leg.
3. Effleurage must not be used over a recent wound or surgical incision
    where there is the danger of stretching the new scar tissue.
4. Effleurage on the body of a very hairy patient may be contra-indicated
    because of the irritating discomfort and the possibility of causing a rash.
    (Some therapists have reported that using a vegetable or nut based
    oil is most helpful with very hairy patients).
5. Massage is not advisable in acute inflammatory conditions,
    e.g. acute arthritis, acute neuritis.

6.   Certain conditions of neuritis or neuralgia, where massage could irritate or aggravate the patient should be avoided.
7.   Massage should not be used where there is bacterial inflammation.
8.   Massage can be used above the site of an acutely inflamed area or over a very recent injury but, once the inflammation has subsided, effleurage may be used over the area itself.

Petrissage

Petrissage is quite different to effleurage and, again, the student must practise over a period of time to become expert. The word is derived from the French meaning to mash or knead with the hands.

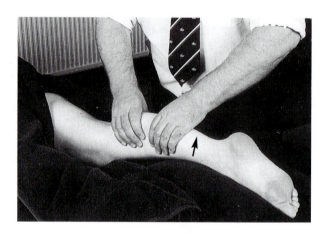

► *Figure 5*
Petrissage of the lower leg.

The principal movement is that of picking up or lifting of the muscles. The muscles are picked or lifted with the hollow of the palm(s) of the hand in a series of rhythmic movements:

Firstly, a simple lifting of the muscle off the bone (or underlying structure). Grasp the muscle with either or both hands, lift and hold with the palmar surface of the hand(s) for a few seconds and then allow the muscle to settle back into position. The easiest muscles to practise on are the posterior muscles of the leg with the patient in a prone position on the plinth. Care should be taken not to nip or pinch the patient by gripping too firmly or, in contrast, the fingers and thumb should not slide towards each other. The aim is to lift and stretch the muscles as far away from the bone as possible.

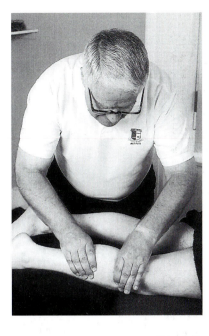

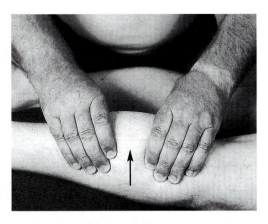

◄ ▲ *Figure 6*
Grasping and lifting
of the muscle.

The next movement is to lift the muscle as before and this time gently but firmly squeeze the muscle belly applying the pressure in the direction of venous return for several seconds before allowing the muscle to settle back into place. This may be repeated a number of times depending upon what the therapist wishes to achieve and, of course, the state of the patient's muscles.

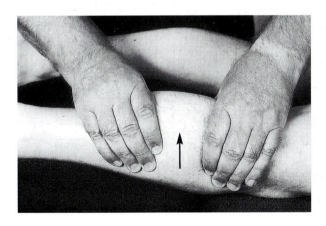

◄ *Figure 7*
Lifting and squeezing
of the muscle.

The next movement of the petrissage cycle is to lift and then roll the muscle away with the thumbs and then back with the fingers. It is important that the underlying tissue be lifted and rolled rather than allowing the fingers and thumbs to merely slide over the surface of the skin. Again, this movement may be performed a number of times during this phase of the treatment depending upon what the therapist wishes to achieve.

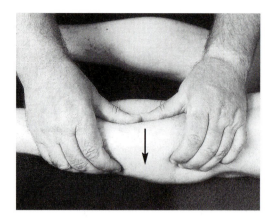

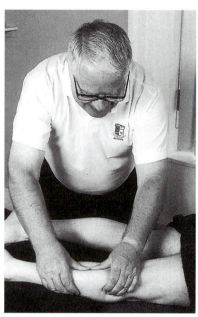

▲ ▶ *Figure 8*
Rolling the muscle.

This is followed by perhaps the best known of the petrissage movements, that of kneading the muscle. The hands are placed on alternate sides of the limb, again the palms of the hands being in full contact with the part being treated. A downward pressure is applied (as opposed to the lifting techniques already described) and a circular movement carried out, the part being kneaded beneath the hands, the hands either moving in the same or opposite directions.

Uneven pressure is applied, or rather the pressure varies during the application of kneading, this pressure again being most when at the furthest point from the heart during the circular movement and lessening at the uppermost part of the circle.

The final movement is that of wringing the muscles. The muscles, having been firmly picked up in both hands are wrung out in much the same way that one applies the wringing of a chamois leather. Wringing is performed on large muscle groups, e.g. calf, gluteals, thigh muscles, obliques and trapezius across the shoulders.

A skilled massage therapist will be able to move their hands quickly and efficiently, alternating with one hand picking up the muscle between palm and thumb and the fingers of the other hand acting on the muscle at the same time.

Petrissage is an important part of remedial massage. The muscles are lifted and manipulated gently but firmly and by the alternate squeezing and relaxing of the pressure, the veins and lymphatic vessels are emptied and filled. The pressure applied, the number of times each movement is repeated, the speed of the movements are all a matter of judgement for the therapist.

Petrissage will help drain metabolic wastes from the tissues and draw in oxygenated blood. Effleurage is then applied to flush the waste products back into the circulatory system.

Along with other measures, Woodward (1967) drew attention to claims that petrissage may be of value in slimming, especially when applied to fatty deposits around the thigh and shoulder regions. His personal experience was that as a result of a really vigorous and energetic massage, the massage therapist is more likely to lose more weight than the client.

Benefits of Petrissage

1. Increases blood flow.
2. Helps flush out waste and reduces local swelling.
3. Loosens adhesions.
4. Improves nutrition to muscle.
5. Relaxes the muscle.
6. A stimulating effect on the nervous system.
7. Reduces pains and aches.

Contra-indications to Petrissage

Petrissage is contra-indicated over inflamed areas and abdominal petrissage is contra-indicated where there is abdominal inflammation such as gastroenteritis or appendicitis; in cases of hernia; during menstruation or pregnancy.

Friction

The first type of friction encountered in remedial massage is a circular movement performed by either the thumb(s) or fingers. This is a deep circular movement applied to muscles and around joints. For example, in back massage, frictions are applied by both thumbs simultaneously from ilium up to the cervical level. It consists of a deep circular friction on the muscles lateral to the spinous processes. Another fruitful area for treatment by frictions is that of the muscular attachments to the scapulae.

Friction generates heat in the tissues, dilates capillaries and increases circulation. Friction breaks down adhesions in and between tissues and around joints. It is one of the therapist's major tools in treating patients with adhesions.

The use of frictions has its pitfalls for the therapist. Wrongly applied or too frequently applied, especially in the early days of training or in practice, may leave a legacy of pain and loss of movement as the joint at the base of the thumb degenerates under the stress of treating patients.

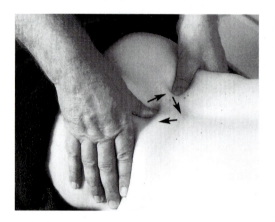

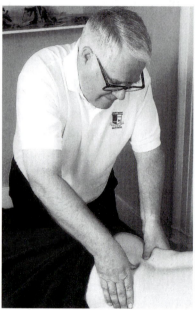

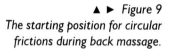

▲ ► *Figure 9*
The starting position for circular frictions during back massage.

A mistake often made by many is that when performing circular friction along a patient's spine, for example, the therapist remains stationary. As the frictions progress towards the cervical region, the therapist remains rooted to the spot and has to stretch and strain to apply the frictions and maintain the same pressure. This puts the pressure more and more on the therapist's thumbs, when a small adjustment of the therapist's feet would allow a much more efficient performance of the friction movements, with the therapist relying more on body weight to get the correct amount of pressure.

Other types and variations of friction are encountered, particularly crossfibre or transverse frictions and logitudinal frictions.

Crossfibre frictions are commonly used at the site of an injury by some therapists and moderate to heavy pressure is used as the fingers move across the tissue. Much is attributed to crossfibre friction almost to the exclusion of any other massage movements, by some of its advocates. It can be quite effective in the treatment of soft tissue, i.e. muscle, tendon and ligament injuries but should be used in conjunction with other massage techniques.

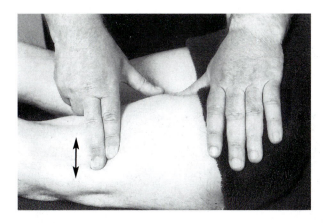

◄ *Figure 10*
Crossfibre friction to the
lateral hamstring tendon.

Hungerford (1991) differentiated between crossfibre and deep transverse friction. Crossfibre frictions, she stated, are applied transversely to the longitude of the muscle fibre at a 90° angle.

Deep transverse friction is a crossfibre stroke given with more depth and more directional emphasis. She claimed it as a superior tool for working with soft tissue injuries. To apply the stroke, the therapist rubs a thumb or finger across the exact site of the lesion (which is determined by functional assessment and palpation). Pressure is less important than a broadening, spreading sense and it is important that the tissue be under proper tension. To treat:

1. Muscles – relaxed to allow deep penetration.
2. Tendons – in the most accessible position.
3. Ligaments – move in one direction and back to simulate normal movement.
4. Sheathed tendons – tendon on a stretch.

Tapotement

Tapotement techniques are used for a stimulating effect and these techniques have been described as a series of brisk blows. An alternative term of description is *'percussion'* meaning *'a striking'*.

Interestingly, Salvo wrote of the derivation from both French and Anglo-Saxon. The Anglo-Saxon word *'taeppa'* means to *'tap'* in the sense of draining fluid from a cavity and, as Salvo pointed out, the mechanical impact of tapotement techniques is still used in some respiratory treatments to loosen congestion in the lungs.

When performed by a skilled and experienced remedial massage therapist, the movements of tapotement are a pleasure to watch. New students often find the techniques difficult and cannot get the hands to work in synchrony. Practise is required and, in the past, many practitioners have literally spent hours practising on cushions placed across their laps whilst sitting in an armchair watching television. There are variations and refinements to the techniques of tapotement in addition to the types described below.

The secret of all tapotement movements is that the action must come from the wrist, rather than from the elbows. Shoulders and elbows remain still and the movements should be practiced by tucking the elbows into the side of the body to prevent them from moving.

Ideally, the hands should never be lifted more than an inch or so off the body of the patient, otherwise the rapid rhythmic performance is impossible. All tapotement techniques should be performed from the wrist with the hands kept in close proximity to the client's body; quite different to many of the illustrations in some of the current books about massage.

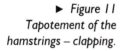
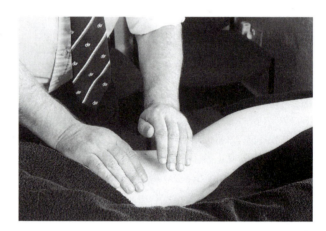

▶ *Figure 11*
Tapotement of the
hamstrings – clapping.

Perhaps the easiest of the movements for the novice is that of clapping. It is done with the palms downward and the fingers extended but forming a hollow curve. The sound of correctly applied clapping is a hollow and deep toned one and not the sharp smacking sound that would be the effect of slapping with the fingers and palm held stiff.

It is quite possible to tell the quality of a therapist's tapotement without having sight of the treatment table but by listening from the next room. Moreover, correctly applied, clapping will not hurt however quickly the therapist is working. Slapping, however, does hurt.

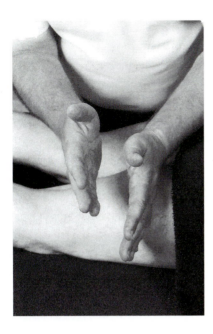
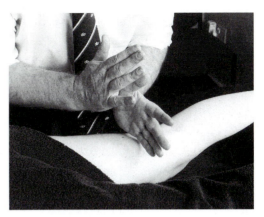

◄ ▲ *Figure 12*
Tapotement of the hamstrings
– hacking – using the ulnar
edge of the hands.

The second movement of tapotement is hacking which is performed with the ulnar border of the hands. The hands are held with the palms facing each other and the thumbs uppermost. Again, the movements are done from the wrist and again this requires constant practise to achieve the rhythmic quick flicking of the wrist in an up-and-down motion.

Viewed in slow motion it is noticeable that the edge of the hands come into contact with the patient's body first and, as the hands flick over, so the edge of the little finger completes the percussion. The experienced therapist is able to angle the hands towards each other so that the same spot on the patient's body is struck by each hand in rapid succession.

Flicking is a very similar movement to hacking except that the edge of the hand is not used, only the fingers. This results in a much lighter application than the hacking movement.

Both beating and pounding are performed with the hands in the closed position. The hands should be relaxed and not tightly clenched. The movement can be performed with the ulnar border of the closed hand (beating) or with the palmar surface of the hands (pounding) moving in rapid succession.

Flailing is referred to in older texts and is a movement similar to clapping except that instead of the palmar surface of the hand being used, the hands are used palms uppermost (again in a relaxed position) and the patient is struck with the backs of the fingers.

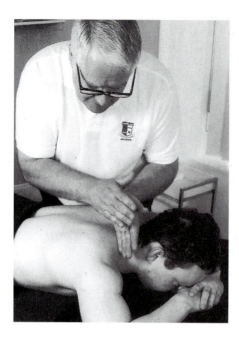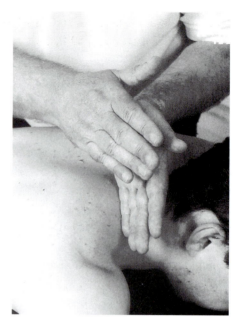

▲ *Figure 13*
Tapotement – flicking with fingers on the trapezius.

Vibration and shaking, though perhaps not truly movements of tapotement, can be introduced here and are often used after tapotement because of their stimulating effects. Tappan, however, described vibration as a fine tremulous movement often used for a soothing effect and noted its use in the treatment of peripheral neuritis and poliomyelitis.

In vibration, the muscle is held lightly in one hand or both hands with the palmar surface of the hand on the limb or body and the entire muscle is rapidly shaken. This needs to be performed very quickly and it is a movement that requires a lot of practise to achieve the desired effect. The movement may be either gentle or vigorous and the effect is similar to that produced by an electrical vibrator.

Vibration has had many claims made on its behalf but is difficult to perform effectively and there is a case for the use of a mechanical or electric vibrator for therapists who are not confident in their own competence.

Benefits of Tapotement

Tapotement is a stimulating movement that causes muscles to contract and draws blood to the skin. It is used to induce muscle tone and there are claims that when used over fleshy parts of the body, such as the thighs and gluteal areas where there are often fatty deposits or flabby areas, tapotement will have a toning effect.

Some authorities, for example Salvo, believe that tapotement has similar effects, but created manually, to ultrasound which has been, in turn, referred to for many years as a *'micromassage'*.

We have already mentioned the role of tapotement in respiratory treatments where it aids in decongesting the lungs by loosening and mobilising phlegm in the respiratory tract.

Contra-indications to Tapotement

Tapotement movements should only be performed over the larger muscle areas of the body and not over bony prominences, superficial nerves, paralysed muscle or in any condition of neurasthenia.

Tapotement may be applied over the abdomen but with caution and restricted to clapping. The heavier movements of beating and pounding should not be applied and are more suitable to the larger muscle groups only. Nor should tapotement be applied to the inner surface of the top of the thigh, the femoral triangle.

Tapotement, because of its stimulating and warming effect is usually applied to healthy bodies rather than in the day-to-day work of the remedial massage therapist who deals with more specific injury situations. Therapists who work with sports people find ample scope for tapotement in their work, especially in the pre-event massage area, rather than in post-event massage where tapotement would be inappropriate.

Compression

I first became aware of the use of compression from watching the techniques of Dr. Myk Hungerford of the Sports Massage Training Institute in California. She used compression in her pre-event massage procedure that is designed to have the athlete functioning at one hundred per cent just prior to an event.

Compression is the rhythmic pumping of the muscle belly and only the muscle belly. Hungerford (1991) described the stroke as a compression, delivered to the belly of the muscle by the palm of the hand and emphasised that the heel of the hand must not be used. The aim of compression is to create hyperaemia which initiates muscle relaxation and releases acetylcholine (the main neurotransmitter of muscle action) and histamines. In her description of pre-event sports massage for the trapezius, Hungerford recommends fifteen compressions in the belly of the muscle alternated with crossfibre frictions to the various attachments. The recommended pressure is about ten pounds per square inch.

How does the therapist find the correct pressure? Stan Duncombe of the Tiny Tim Centre in Coventry used to resort to bathroom scales when teaching the correct pressure for neuromuscular techniques. Try using your hands on bathroom scales to record the correct pressure.

Lubricant is not necessary as the pressure is applied perpendicularly to the patient. I used a series of techniques based on Hungerford's movements in rather unusual circumstances. Some years ago, I accompanied an eight-man team on a long-distance relay from Lands End to John O'Groats. There was one runner on the road for one hour at any one time. The team members ran for an hour and then had seven hours rest before the next run. I accompanied the squad to give massage treatments and my mobile treatment room was the back of an estate car (which I also had to drive).

Not the place for bottles of oil or treatment tables or for the full remedial massage routines of effleurage and petrissage. I applied compression and muscle belly pressure techniques with crossfibre frictions and some mobilisations. The runners responded well and all eight completed their eight hundred-odd miles of running without injury.

Compression is not merely to be used in pre-event sports massage and is usefully employed by many therapists in other circumstances, particularly in association with approximation. This is a technique of applying compression above and below the site of discomfort, maintain the compression and bring the hands towards each other. This movement brings the ends of the muscle being compressed towards each other.

Nerve Stroke

I am always a little intrigued when perusing the test papers of our Canadian students who are taught by Joyce Raiwet at her centre in Clyde, Alberta. They always make some reference to the 'Nerve Stroke' as the finishing touch to their massage procedure.

The nerve stroke is a very light stroking movement at the end of a treatment, a very light effleurage. It is done slowly and lightly to whichever part of the body has just been treated and it has a soothing effect on the nervous system.

This is not to be confused with a more specific nerve stroke applied to the distribution of the sciatic nerve. After whatever treatment the therapist feels justified, the therapist finishes the treatment by stroking from the small of the back, down the back of each leg. Each stroke travels a little further down towards the heel. Again, a light but steady pressure is applied with the aim of soothing the irritated sciatic nerve.

Sports Massage

Remedial massage is an excellent foundation upon which to base a career in sports massage or the treatment of sports men and women. Consider the injury situation alone. Briggs (2000) highlighted a Sports Council report of 1998 that considered thirteen sports and identified nineteen million sports injuries a year with 1.4 million serious enough to keep the athlete off work for an average of six days. These statistics alone imply that there is a need for therapists to assist in the recovery from these injuries.

In the minds of many therapists, the role of remedial massage in sport is very much that of the treatment of injuries. It is an extension of the old idea of, "My legs feel a bit stiff, let's have a rub down." This is but one side of the equation – the treatment of the after-effects of taking part in sport, the casualties.

Massage has other roles to play. Among others, Lachman (1988) and Hungerford (1993) listed a range of benefits of massage to sports people including:

- Speeds recovery-time during intense training and helps the athlete train without discomfort.
- Aids in the prevention of injuries.
- Helps the athlete to train in an injury-free environment.
- Assists in keeping a primary injury from becoming a secondary injury.
- Helps eliminate stress and tension during training and pre-competition.
- Helps the athlete maintain a consistent training schedule.
- Generally lengthens an athlete's career.
- Helps improve performance during competition.

Much of the evidence for Hungerford's claims is anecdotal. However, the anecdotal evidence is quite weighty and comes not only from weekend club athletes but from Olympic champions and many top class professional sports people. As well as the physical effects of massage for sports people, one should not underestimate the psychological effects mentioned in the Olympic Book of Sports Medicine (1988).

Sports massage, though used in ancient times in the amphitheatre, was undoubtedly practiced but little known and unorganised in the Western world until the Olympic Games of 1972 when Lasse Viren won gold medals in two events, the 5000 and 10000 metres races. He claimed that the secret of his success was daily massage. From that point on there was a growing interest in massage for sports people in America, centred on the definitive book by Meagher called, 'Sports Massage'. From America the interest in sports massage has spread worldwide.

Dr. M. Hungerford, is a leading advocate of sports massage in America and is widely credited with having massage accepted as an official part of the Medical Command of the Olympic programme for the 1984 Olympic Games. She defined sports massage as the application of massage techniques to enhance athletic performance. Sports massage encompasses pre-event and post-event, during competition, pre-race and post-race, during training and conditioning and, perhaps the phase with which remedial massage therapists are more familiar, restoration-rehabilitation for both acute and chronic injuries.

In pre-event massage the aim is to enhance muscular tone and flexibility to prepare the athlete for competition. The pre-event massage is not used instead of the warm-up, mobilising and stretching routine, as Lachman appeared to think. Pre-event massage is used in conjunction with these other activities to prepare the athlete in that forty-five or fifty minute period immediately prior to competition. Nor is pre-event so much of a luxury as it was fifteen years ago; there are now many trained personnel in many areas of sport available through clubs and associations to provide pre- and post-event massage.

Post-event massage seeks to create a prolonged state of reduced muscular tension and to fend off delayed onset muscle soreness (DOMS). By applying massage during training and conditioning, for example in pre-season training, the athlete trains without aches and pains which helps them train more consistently without injury.

The restoration and rehabilitation, whether dealing with acute or chronic injury, helps the athlete return to sport more quickly and with less discomfort. Along with the skills of massage and the ability to apply these skills to achieve different ends, the sports massage practitioner requires other attributes:

* A sound knowledge of anatomy and physiology.
* The ability to evaluate musculoskeletal tone and determine strength and condition of athletes.
* An understanding of the principles of training and conditioning.
* An understanding of the coaching and training methods used.

- An ability to exhibit an acute understanding of muscle, joint mobility and biomechanics, pertinent to the individual athlete.
- A comprehensive understanding of the athlete's sport.

An interesting insight into this subject has been supplied directly to me by several massage therapists currently employed by professional soccer clubs in both England and Scotland. The awareness of the value of massage in its various forms, for example pre- and post-event massage, has risen sharply to coincide with the increasing numbers of foreign professionals. Michael Greener, the massage therapist at Newcastle United reported in lecture (1998) that when he started to give massage treatments at Newcastle, the players were suspicious and sceptical and did not come forward for treatment. Rather they attended the two physiotherapists on the staff for the 'traditional' treatments by exercise and electrotherapy. Newcastle United signed David Ginola, a French international who regarded massage treatment as part of his daily routine as a professional footballer. David became a regular patient for pre-event, post-event and inter-event massage.

This at first intrigued the native-born players and when they saw how well Ginola performed they began to turn up at the massage table with a request to Michael, "Give us a Ginola."

Top soccer players from Italy, France, Germany and Holland have arrived in the UK expecting to have massage treatments on a daily basis as part of their training and conditioning programme to enable them to continue to play injury free and meet the demands of our professional season.

Sports massage and therapy is a booming area of massage with many therapists seeking to establish themselves as successful practitioners. A thorough training in remedial massage is an excellent preparation for such a career.

Pre-event Massage

The aims of pre-event massage are, stated Hungerford (1998), to promote speed, power, endurance and to prevent injury to the athlete. Pre-event massage is given to help prepare the athlete physically and mentally for better performance.

The best time to give pre-event massage to the athlete is within the four hours preceding the event (Benjamin and Lamp, 1996) with the optimum time, suggested by Hungerford, during the warm-up phase, i.e. between forty-five and fifteen minutes prior to taking part in sporting activity. This confirmed King's (1993) earlier recommendation that the massage take place between thirty to forty-five minutes before competing and should be of fifteen to twenty minutes duration and as an adjunct to the warm-up.

The essence of pre-event massage is deep repetitive compressions to the belly of a muscle, with transverse friction to the attachments of the muscles, i.e. the origins and insertions. The general format is of three sets of compressions alternated with three sets of crossfibre frictions at the origins and insertions of the muscles. However, this should be varied according to the individual requirements of the athlete.

In applying the compressions, the technique is to apply the palm of one hand while the hands are in the palmar-overlay position (one hand on top of the other). The hands are positioned in the centre or belly of the muscle and the pressure is applied directly downwards.

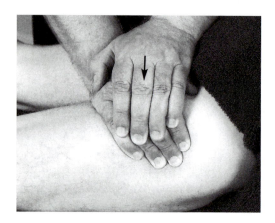

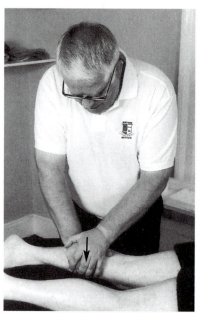

▲ ▶ *Figure 14*
Sports massage – pre-event –
compression to the muscle belly.

The compressions should be administered rhythmically and progressively deeper with each set. The massage should be deep to be effective but take care not to cause pain to the athlete. Depth can be obtained by progression. This form of massage must only be given to strong, healthy persons; it is too powerful to give to the frail, the elderly and the already injured.

Compressions

The muscle is compressed in the belly by the palm of the hand in what Hungerford described as a rhythmic 'sucking' motion. This technique, correctly applied, performs several functions including spreading the muscle fibres and intensifying blood supply in the muscle.

Crossfibre Frictions

Crossfibre frictions are applied by the finger tips or the thumb. There is a possibility of some local soreness but the longer-term effects outweigh any possible short-term soreness. Local crossfibre strokes to connective tissue generally leave no soreness. The therapist applies three firm strokes to each origin and insertion, again with a steady rhythmic flow.

The purposes of the crossfibre frictions are to loosen scar tissue and adhesions that may exist in the tendons and sheathing, to re-align damaged fibres, to render scar tissue more pliable and less likely to irritate surrounding tissues. The frictions accomplish this by helping create what Hungerford described as a fibrillory network within the scar tissue itself. Again, it should be noted that these techniques should not be used on new injuries. King warned against the strong use of crossfibre frictions in pre-event massage, especially on athletes who were not used to receiving massage treatment; anything that is painful to the athlete will detract from performance rather than enhance it.

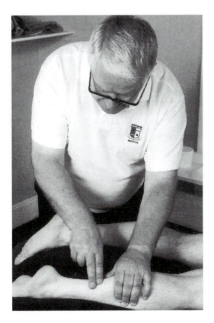

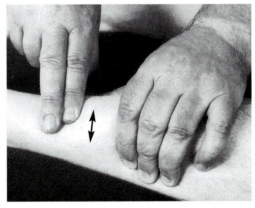

◄ ▲ *Figure 15*
Crossfibre frictions to the Achilles tendon.

We tend to think of sports massage as an invention of modern times. In their excellent book, Benjamin and Lamp reproduced descriptions of both pre- and post-event massage from the writings of Galen (130 – 200 AD). Galen, a Greek physician in Rome, for a period of time was physician and surgeon to the gladiators and described in detail the procedure for tripsis paraskeuastike (i.e. massage before exercise). He described both compression and friction techniques and how they can be used to, *"excite it (the body) to activity and augment its tone."*

A Pre-event Sequence for Legs and Hips

The emphasis of pre-event massage should be on the major muscle groups that will be used in the actual event. Thus, for athletics the emphasis may be on the legs and hips:

Gluteals

Compressions to gluteus maximus and medius and piriformis.
Transverse frictions to origins and insertions of maximus and medius.
Transverse frictions across humeral insertion of piriformis.
3 sets

Legs

Compressions to hamstrings.
Deep transverse frictions to origins and insertions of hamstrings.
Compressions to gastrocnemius and soleus.
Transverse frictions to Achilles tendon.
3 sets

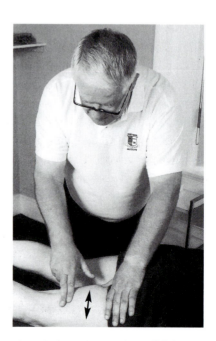

▶ *Figure 16*
Crossfibre frictions to the
lateral hamstrings tendon.

Foot

Thumb compressions to plantar surface.
Transverse frictions to metatarsal heads.
Transverse frictions across origin of plantar fascia at calcaneum.
3 sets

Legs

Compressions of quadriceps and tensor fasciae latae.
Transverse frictions of origins of rectus femoris, sartorius and tensor fasciae latae.
3 sets

The effects of a pre-event massage given in this manner should be to:

1. Improve cellular nutrition through dilation of capillaries caused
    by the deep rhythmic compressions;
2. Break up adhesions by the deep transverse frictions;
3. Improve function of tendons and ligaments thus increasing flexibility;
4. Release trigger points;
5. Remove hypertonicity in the muscles;
6. Provide an opportunity for relaxation and anxiety reduction
    and also to mentally focus on the impending event.

All of this should result in the athlete achieving peak performance with reduced risk of injuries.

Areas of the Body Where Special Care is Required

All massage therapists are acquainted with areas of the body where a little extra care and vigilance is required. Not every one agrees with all the areas or the degree of care required. I recall a very recent discussion with the redoubtable Grace Halliday, the Deep Lymphatic therapist from South Australia, about the pressure to be used in the popliteal area. Grace was of the opinion that students did not use enough pressure when working in this area. Students are taught to ease off with the pressure of the massage strokes when approaching the popliteal space that contains the popliteal aertery. The effects of working in this part of the body would differ enormously depending on whether the therapist is an (almost) untutored student or a therapist with over fifty years clinical experience like Grace Halliday.

The capacity for harm remains, however, and all therapists must be aware of certain structures, tissues, areas of the human body that are more liable to injury.

Nicely described by Salvo as "endangerment sites" they are areas containing certain anatomical structures that may be damaged by direct or sustained pressures applied during a massage treatment.

Nerve compression may cause loss of motor control, pain or numbness. Pressure on vascular vessels may cause bleeding, bruising or affect blood flow. Pressure on organs may cause pain, nausea or even dysfunction. Care must be taken when treating by massage in the following areas:

- The femoral triangle.
- The popliteal space.
- The axilla.
- The anterior neck and the brachial area.
- Around the ears.
- Around the throat.
- The elbow, especially the medial epicondyle.
- The distribution of the sciatic nerve.
- The spinous processes.
- The ribs, especially the floating ribs.
- The breasts.
- Avoid any lymph node when enlarged.
- The eyes especially avoid any direct pressure to the eyeball.

About Muscles and Joints

Hundreds of muscles are involved in the range of human movement and they act in inter-related groups of functional units rather than as separate entities, for example the quadriceps group and hamstring group working to produce flexion and extension at the knee.

Each movable joint has its certain normal range of movements within which its action is smooth, free and unrestricted. There are many pathological conditions that can cause limitation of movement within joints. Some of these conditions will respond to massage and manipulation – others will definitely not. Where movement is restricted because of new fibrous tissue or adhesions that have formed in or around the joint or in the muscles that act upon it, many of these cases respond exceptionally well to massage.

A simple movable joint consists of two or more articular surfaces covered with cartilage and enclosed in a fibrous capsule. The capsule is lined by the synovial membrane that secretes synovial fluid into the joint. This fluid acts as a carrier of nutrients and as a lubricant for the joint. Small fat deposits are found within the

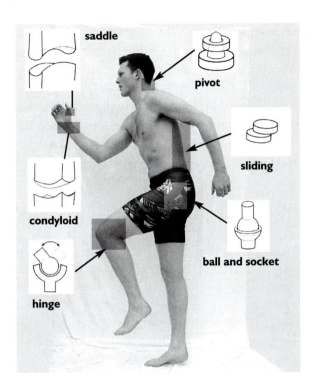

saddle

pivot

sliding

condyloid

ball and socket

hinge

◄ Figure 17
Some of the
different joints
found in the body.

joint which fill up the gaps between the bone articulations and thus there are no empty spaces within the joint. A good example of an incongruent joint is the knee where tibia and femur do not fit snugly together like two pieces of a jigsaw.

Ligaments are tough and inelastic and their function is to control the range of movement and prevent extremes of movement and joint displacement or dislocation. The ligaments become taut when a joint is taken to the full extent of its range of movement and beyond. Injury to a ligament, usually in which, perhaps, a few of the fibres tear, is referred to as a sprain.

A sprain is an abnormal wrenching of a joint. This can be very painful and is aggravated by any movement that places strain upon the ligament. Other tissues around the joint may also be injured at the time the injury is sustained. There will also be tenderness on palpation over the site of the injury and there will be swelling around the joint, though this may vary depending upon the overall damage inflicted on the joint and its tissues. An injury leads to loss of tone and atrophy of the muscles that act upon the joint. This atrophy occurs very quickly and can be quite a significant factor in recovery.

Adhesions may form around the joint as the result of the sprain and may become chronic resulting in discomfort, pain upon certain movements, and a reduction in the range of movement at the joint.

When a joint is injured, the muscles that act upon that joint are always affected and the therapist should ensure that treatment is not directed to the joint alone. The muscles must also be treated for the patient to attain a good recovery.

Muscle grouping in relation to movement and posture is an important one for therapists to keep in mind, when performing examinations and planning treatments. Muscle dysfunction occurring in one muscle will affect the whole group of muscles and have knock-on effects to other groups of muscles.

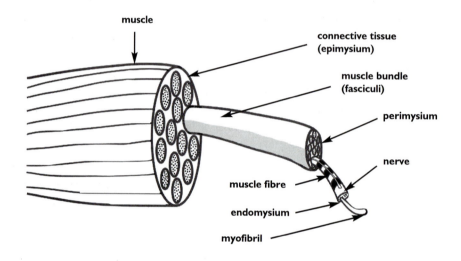

▲ *Figure 18*
A cross-section of skeletal muscle.

The muscles involved in shoulder movements provide a good example since many muscles are involved in shoulder movements and each movement at the shoulder involves more than one muscle. We must therefore take into consideration all the muscles associated with shoulder movement when examining and treating a patient with shoulder dysfunction. As other muscles of the shoulder become involved in the effects of the injury, the original dysfunction may be masked and the patient may present with different symptoms and contractions in muscles from those originally affected by the strain.

Pain that occurs when performing a movement, may be caused by the concentric action of the muscles used to carry out the movements, i.e. the agonists; it may also be caused by stretching out of the abnormally contracted antagonists.

Body movement is most efficient when the musculoskeletal system is in balance, for example, we take getting out of bed each morning for granted but it is a very painful experience if the person has a spasm of the spinal muscles. The spine is in the centre of the back and is held in place by a series of muscles and ligaments. Uneven muscular development may upset the balance and pull the spine out of alignment causing a scoliosis. This may be caused by abnormal muscular contraction or excessive muscular development on one side of the spine, perhaps due to many years of poor posture when performing tasks at work.

For some athletes, for example, tennis players, unevenness of muscle development may be hard to avoid. It is a common occurrence in the workplace where repetitive actions over a period of time may not only produce an imbalance in muscular development but may lead on to what has become known as repetitive strain injury (RSI).

An imbalance may develop within a group of muscles and cause symptoms of pain, loss of strength and function. It is interesting to compare the relative development of vastus medialis in many 'joggers' and their more explosive fellow athletes, the sprinters. Different demands on the muscles, particularly vastus medialis, lead to a very different pattern of development. Sprinters tend to develop bigger muscles in the quadriceps group, especially vastus medialis. Among 'joggers' a less well-developed vastus medialis may cause an imbalance between it and the other muscles in the group. This imbalance may affect the functioning of the patella during knee flexion and extension, that may cause pain when running.

Muscle balance must be considered in cases where the muscles performing certain actions are stronger than their antagonists. Quadriceps are stronger than hamstrings and many injuries occur in sport when the leg is suddenly and rapidly extended by the stronger quadriceps muscles and the antagonistic hamstrings are injured by the sudden and violent movement. Perhaps they are unprepared for the movement, fatigued, or not warmed-up.

Muscular imbalance may also occur in a limb that has been injured and there has been a compensatory use of the uninjured side that may put strain on the good limb. The overworked limb should receive the attention of the therapist as well as the injured one. Failure to do so will result in dysfunction of the uninjured leg and possible chronic injury.

Some muscle groups may abnormally shorten due to overuse. This may happen, for example, in some of the postural muscles that, because of their actions, may have a greater tendency to develop abnormal contraction than some other muscles. Postural muscles that are prone to abnormal contraction include the calf muscle, hamstrings, iliopsoas, gluteals, erector spinae and pectorals. The abnormal contractions make the muscles concerned much less efficient and more prone to injury.

Postural muscles take more continuous strain but tend not to move as rapidly as other muscles. They have more endurance and are in a state of tonus all the time, except during sleep when they refresh and repair themselves. Sleep and rest are very important as part of the treatment of injured postural muscles.

The postural activity of muscles is under the control of reflex nervous action and as such is influenced by the central nervous system. Causes of postural deficiency are neurological, either general or local, noted by Woodward (1967). Common causes include:

- Neurasthenia.
- Mental fatigue.
- Inertia due to worry or overwork.
- Nervous debility following illness.

Pain can inhibit postural activity of muscles – already mentioned earlier, that sprained joints are often accompanied by loss of tone in the muscles acting upon the joint. A good example is the loss of tone and atrophy of the quadriceps following injury to the knee. Another often quoted example is that of a person who has a leg in plaster for six or eight weeks following a fracture and the obvious visual differences between the injured leg and the healthy leg upon removal of the plaster.

It is mentioned in the section about examination of the patient, that one of the questions the therapist should ask each patient is that of sleep disturbance caused by the injury. If the patient is having disturbed sleep due to the symptoms of the injury, the probability is that the recovery process will be slow until the sleep pattern improves. Sleep is a natural aid to healing and recovery.

When formulating a treatment plan, the therapist must take in to consideration the question of muscle balance. Massage treatment alone may not be sufficient and stretching, mobilising and strengthening activities will become important aspects of the treatment regime for most patients.

Skeletal Muscle Tone

Muscle tone is the term used to describe the amount of tautness that is present in skeletal muscle at rest. The slight coupling of cross-bridges which is present even in relaxed muscle, helps keep the body in correct posture and allows muscle contraction to commence more easily. This residual degree of contraction in skeletal muscle is essential for many other normal body functions, such as holding the eyes open and the jaw closed.

It is thought that skeletal muscle tone results from nerve impulses originating partly from the brain and partly by reflex action via the spinal cord, as the constant stretching of the muscles between their attachments stimulates the muscle spindles. If spindle impulses are blocked, the muscle normally loses all tone and becomes flaccid.

Muscle tone is greater in those muscle groups responsible for maintaining posture such as the extensor group of the lower limbs, the trunk and the head. Postural tone helps maintain the equilibrium and stability of the joints.

The degree of muscle tone will vary depending upon the amount of exercise to which the muscle is subjected. Exercise of a particular muscle group will lead to an increase in strength and muscle tone, while weak muscles will have less tone.

Normal muscle tone is the normal state of the muscle at rest, with only a few muscle fibres stimulated. Muscles may reflect more tension, an abnormal state of muscular contraction, which will, however, usually return to its normal tonal state.

The abnormal state of muscle contraction may persist, the muscle become hypertonic and may show signs of injury. The muscles may require treatment to help restore normal muscle tone.

An abnormal state of muscle contraction may not only result in muscle injury but will affect the joint or joints upon which the muscle works, resulting in loss of function at the joint. At its worst, the abnormal state of muscle contraction is referred to as a 'spasm' or 'cramp', which is very painful and will require treatment to return the muscles to their normal state.

Atrophy

Atrophy is a diminution in the size of muscles and may be caused by:

*   Immobilisation and subsequent impaired metabolism.
*   Injury or disease of joints – as well as immobilisation,
    nerve damage can cause inhibition of activity of cells in muscle fibres.
*   Pressure reduces blood supply and impairs function.
*   Circulatory disturbance – a lack of circulation means a gradual
    decrease in nutrition and loss of size of the muscle.
*   Disorders of the nervous system affect muscle and lead to atrophy.

Blood Supply

Muscles have a network of blood vessels averaging some three thousand per cubic millimetre. At rest some ninety-five per cent of these are closed down as surplus to requirements for the level of functioning of the body.

During activity these blood vessels open to demand and ensure that there is a sufficient supply of blood to the working fibres and the transport of 'used' blood away from the muscles.

During vigorous effort, more and more of the vessels are employed and the flow increases from fifteen per cent of cardiac output to something like seventy-two per cent of cardiac output going to muscles.

Flexibility

Flexibility in human movement is the capacity to twist, turn or bend, allowing the joints to move through their full range of movements without causing intrinsic injury.

It is often assumed that merely using muscles creates flexibility but skeletal muscles must also be 'stretched' in order to maintain flexibility and allow maximal range of movement. Any recreational or occupational pursuits in which muscles are repeatedly contracted may cause the muscles to shorten, thereby reducing flexibility. Repeated contraction of a muscle will produce abnormal muscle contraction. This reduces flexibility and places stress on joints, muscles, tendons, ligaments and connective tissue. This lack of flexibility due to abnormal muscular contraction will increase the possibility of muscle injury.

Flexibility can be improved and the risk of injury reduced if the extent of abnormal muscle contraction is decreased. It should be emphasised that a flexibility programme is very important in injury prevention. However, there is a tendency to regard flexibility training only as remedial exercise, to be undertaken as part of the recovery programme after injury.

At some joints and in certain movements, for example the elbow, the bony structure will limit movement, however, the major resistance at most joints is provided by soft tissues, e.g. muscles, ligaments and tendons. Muscles and tendons make up much of the resistance to flexibility, such is the part played by abnormal muscle contractions on the flexibility of a joint and massage and stretching are of great value in any flexibility programme.

Muscle and Tendon Injury

Muscles and tendons function together as a unit and an injury to one part of the unit affects the other even though it is uninjured. Injuries may occur in the muscle itself, at the junction of the muscle and tendon, in the tendon or at the tendon's insertion into the bone where there may be an avulsion.

The muscle or tendon may be partially or completely ruptured. Sometimes the injury is caused by compression, the result of impact or trauma, for example where the muscle is crushed between an external object and the bone. Contributing factors to muscle and tendon injury:

- Muscles that are poorly prepared for activity, for example, no warm-up before a sporting event.
- Lack of fitness.
- Weakness caused by previous injury and incomplete recovery from that injury.
- Weakness caused by scar tissue from a previous injury.
- Overstretching the muscle.
- Fatigue which makes the muscle less efficient and more prone to injury; the protective reflexes respond more slowly.
- Tense muscles.
- Exposure to cold that makes a muscle function less efficiently and, as in the case of fatigued muscles, the protective reflexes respond more slowly.
- A mild muscle rupture affects a small percentage of the fibres in a muscle and results in no great loss of strength or restriction of movement; active movement may cause discomfort around the area of damage.
- A moderate rupture causes pain that is aggravated by any attempt to contract the muscle. Thus, movement and posture are affected.
- A total rupture involves disruption of the whole unit. The pain experienced is sharp and severe but recedes with rest. Any attempt to contract the muscle reproduces the severe symptoms. There will be swelling and discolouration.
- The repair is by scar tissue formation. A poor repair has a lot of fibrous tissue that is easily disturbed and may rupture again. The more fibrous tissue there is present, the less efficient the muscle becomes.

Chapter 3
The Therapist in Action

The Patient

First Appearances

The therapist has about fifteen seconds during which period of time, the patient will arrive at a judgement of the therapist. Once the patient has walked into your treatment room, shaken hands with you and taken a seat, your fate may be sealed. The patient likes the look of the therapist, begins to feel confident about the therapist and begins to believe that the therapist will do him some good. Or the opposite may happen.

Reports on research at the University of Toledo led by Professor F. Bernieri and reported in the Daily Mail (15.6.2000) concluded that the handshake was vitally important. The Professor claimed that this research offers proof that you never get a second chance to make a first impression.

The patient's response to the therapist is often 'pre-verbal', i.e. before a word is spoken. The patient notes how the therapist walks through the door, the therapist's posture, whether the therapist has a captivating aura, whether he has a firm, confident handshake. I believe it's often as basic as that. It's what we all know as 'first impressions' and for many people these first impressions are lasting impressions from which they are unlikely to stray.

On one occasion, in my role as an examiner, I 'failed' a student who presented for a practical/oral examination attired in floral shirt, shorts and beach shoes. This was despite the fact that all students are required to dress in clinical attire and are reminded of this on many occasions during the course. As far as I was concerned this student was dressed inappropriately as much for a formal examination, as he would have been in a clinical setting, despite the weather being quite sunny and warm.

I agreed with him that his mode of dress may well have met with the approval of his social peers but certainly would not meet with the approval of the great majority of patients. The patient expects the therapist to look like a professional. When the patient is then put in the position of meeting someone who dresses so inappropriately, a draining of confidence in the therapist soon follows. This opinion was reinforced by Harper (1999) who stated that the therapist should always present a professional appearance to patients.

Manner

The therapist's manner and speech is also of supreme importance; his personality is a crucial factor (Walker, 1995). An unsmiling, monosyllabic therapist does not make a good impression. A welcoming smile, a greeting and a handshake helps put the patient at ease and shapes his or her first impression of the therapist. Many patients who visit for the first time are filled with trepidation and remember half-truths about necks being cracked. The patient may feel exactly the same about visiting you for treatment as some people feel about a visit to the dentist. A welcoming smile and greeting goes a long way to establishing a good patient-therapist relationship.

Alongside dress and manner, the therapist should make sure that the treatment room and its environment is clean, fresh and attractively decorated. Patients will not come to run down and dilapidated rooms and premises. The patient should have a comfortable chair on which to sit. The therapist does not need to spend a lot of money on complete refurbishment but he does need to make sure that his premises and treatment room are as professionally correct as possible.

The patient takes in all of this simultaneously and an impression, for good or bad, is made. On occasions, and quite unprompted by me, some of my patients have told me of their encounters with previous medical professionals right across the spectrum.

These examples included a confrontation with two very excited dogs in the practitioner's waiting room and the unconvincing assurance by the practitioner that "they only want to play". Another practitioner, it was reported only two or three years ago, sat and smoked during the initial interview. Another could not satisfy his appetite and ate his pie and peas with his bare hands in between the various sections of treatment and did not attempt to wash his hands prior to examining the patient. Another kept his ear piece attached during a treatment lest he missed his test match commentary and kept interrupting the treatment with a series of "Ooohs" and "Ahhhs". I felt embarrassed for our profession when told of these incidents by patients who were quite scathing about such practitioners. In the patients' eyes these misdemeanors negated any claims to caring, healing and professionalism.

The image the patient has of a practitioner is very important and the practitioner should take good care about creating the correct image. This extends from the professional to the social life and the personal life of the practitioner. An image that may have taken many years to build up may be wrecked by some momentary action or association away from the treatment room, for example an involvement with a 'fringe' political movement or a prosecution for drunken driving.

Patients expect and desire ordinary human warmth and friendliness and have no wish to be treated with objective blandness. The patient must be able to sense that he is dealing with a real person who will understand their problem and treat them honestly and with openness and respect.

A personal opinion – I do not like to be called by my first name by complete strangers. Firstly, I do not use my first name and, secondly, it presumes a degree of intimacy that is not justified. You just know that the guilty party is parroting the 'training manual' whether they are traffic policemen, hospital clerical workers, health club attendants or the like. I rarely feel any sincerity emanating from these people. Many patients do not like to be called by their first name and certainly not at the initial visit. It often sounds insincere and patronising.

Most middle-aged and elderly patients like and expect to be called, "Mr" or "Mrs" or "Miss". It may be that at some stage during the course of treatments they will tell you to call them by their first name. Fine. I always made it a point of professional courtesy to address patients by title or surname until invited otherwise by the patient. Some patients invite this greater degree of intimacy once they are completely at ease with you and your treatments. It is almost like a battle honour.... you have earned their approval and friendship and not simply taken it for granted.

Note-taking and Record Keeping

Once the patient has arrived for his appointment he should be seen punctually. I hate to be kept waiting when I turn up on time for an appointment and I made a promise when I started out in practice to try my best to prevent this happening to my patients.

Allow plenty of time when meeting patients for the first time. Even to the extent of bringing the patient into the treatment room and sitting the patient down then leaving them in the room for a few seconds so that they can accustom themselves to your clinic. This will allow them to take in the tidy, pleasant professional surroundings and catch a glimpse of your professional diplomas and certificates.

Ideally, therapist and patient sit down and by the artful use of questions the practitioner gets the patient to tell him why he has made the appointment, what condition troubles him, how long has he been suffering and all the relevant information about himself. The key point in this process is that the patient should be encouraged to talk and the therapist should listen.

This is the beginning of the examination process and it should also be the beginning of the healing process, too. If the patient realises that he is being listened to by an understanding and sympathetic professional, who is willing to take time and care, then the patient begins to relax. Relaxation was, according to Hippocrates, the beginning of the healing process.

There will be occasions when the examination procedure will take twenty or thirty minutes. On other occasions there will be a need for some form of treatment to begin fairly quickly and the examination will be of shorter duration.

We have all experienced the constraints and shortcomings of the health service at one time or another in this respect. Patients used to tell me about the 'Triple Two Syndrome' that was supposed to exist in a neighbouring health authority. They reckoned that, if referred to a consultant for a musculoskeletal problem, there was a two-year wait. When your appointment arrived you would have to wait two hours at the hospital to see the consultant. The long-awaited consultation lasted a mere two minutes!

When listening to the patient's account of their injury, resist the urge to write notes as the patient talks. The practitioner must listen to the patient and be seen to be listening. Note-taking is difficult and important pieces of information that the patient tells you will be lost. It is also off-putting to the patient and there is a tendency for the patient to lose concentration and, sometimes, to avoid telling details if they see that everything they say is being written down.

A good time to write notes is during the period of time after your conversation with the patient and when they are undressing behind the screen. If this is not convenient use the time between appointments to write your notes. Do not leave them until the end of a busy day. Either you will be too tired to consider writing your patient notes or you will confuse the patients and their conditions and treatments and enter incorrect information.

Patient records are most important and details of all examinations and treatments must be kept meticulously. Failure to keep records will cause you serious problems sooner rather than later.

An example from my own experience will illustrate this point. A patient came to me for treatment following a road traffic accident in which she had sustained a fairly typical 'whiplash' injury. Upon examination I also found a sacro-iliac injury. I entered my examination finding on her record card and, among others I wrote that she had a left sacro-iliac lesion.

At the next appointment I asked her how she felt including her left lower back. She corrected me and said it was her right lower back. My mistake. I crossed out 'left' and scrawled 'right' above it on the card.

Some five years later a solicitor came to see me from his office, to discuss the forthcoming high court case featuring his client, my patient, who was claiming substantial damages as the result of the road accident.

The solicitor had a problem. It was the patient's record card. He wanted to know who had altered the notes, when were they changed, why was the change not witnessed and dated. My carelessness, he claimed, hindered his client's case and that the opposition would tear my testimony to pieces. It was a chastening experience but fortunately I was not required to appear in the high court on that occasion as the parties reached an out of court settlement two days prior to the court date.

Preparing the Patient for Treatment

Every practitioner should have either a screened changing area or a changing room in which patients can remove clothing prior to examination and treatment and, of course, in which to get dressed again after treatment.

It is unacceptable to have patients remove their clothing in front of the therapist. Each and every patient must be allowed some privacy and must have their modesty treated with respect. Not only must there be adequate changing arrangements but patients must also be given towels to cover their bodies until the time arrives for specific examination or treatment to a specific area of the patient's body.

My patients have, on occasions, told me of some quite dreadful lapses of professional etiquette by practitioners. Of occasions when a new patient has been put in the embarrassing situation of having to disrobe completely under the gaze of a therapist; of being left semi-naked for minutes on end in a room to which other people had access including the window cleaner. At best, patients do not return to practitioners who do not respect their modesty and who cause them such embarrassment. At worst, the patient treated in this way will tell their family and friends and word soon travels about how such a therapist treats his patients.

Hygiene in the Treatment Room

The therapist must follow the rules of hygiene at all times:

- The first essential is the awareness that absolute cleanliness is required at all times.
- The towels must be clean and warmed prior to use.
- Linen or towelling used on the treatment table, e.g. pillowcases, couch covers, must be clean and fresh for each patient.
- Equipment and apparatus, for example the plinth or electrotherapy equipment, must be kept clean and disinfected on occasions.
- Any waste materials must be removed from the treatment room each day and do not allow over-filled rubbish containers to be viewed by patients.
- The room must be warm and well ventilated.
- A clean fresh coat or tunic should be worn each day or more frequently if the weather is very warm or the therapist spills something on the tunic.
- The therapist must wash his hands thoroughly before and after each treatment.
- Hands and nails should be checked daily.
- The therapist should present himself to the patients in a clean and tidy way.
- Wrist watches and jewelry should not be worn because of the dangers of injuring the patient and of harbouring microorganisms which may infect the patient.
- Open containers should not be used for cream or lubricant because of the dangers of cross-infection. Therefore closed, pump-action type containers should be used.
- How safe is the lubricant? Will it cause any adverse reactions in the patients?
- The therapist should not treat patients if he, the therapist, has any illness or an infection.
- You should be able to offer toilet facilities. Are they clean and well ventilated?
- Have animals access to the treatment rooms? Make sure that they have not. There is nothing more off-putting to a patient than an 'animal smell' to greet them as they enter the premises. Tobacco odour is equally repugnant to non-smokers.

- On occasions, the therapist may have the need to wear vinyl gloves during treatment, for example, some aspects of sports injury treatment, or if engaged in manipulative therapy treatment of the temporomandibular joint. Hands must be washed after the removal of the gloves also.
- Therapists must familiarise themselves with Health and Safety rules and regulations relating to their premises and equipment.
- Every therapist should possess current insurance cover relating to their property and equipment and to their patients' safety and well being.

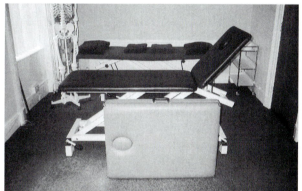

a.

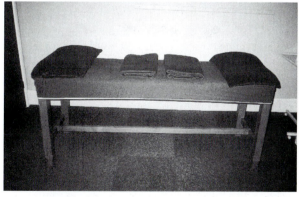

◄ Figure 19
Three different types
of treatment table –
(a) portable plinth;
(b) wooden fixed-
height plinth;
(c) hydraulic plinth.

b.

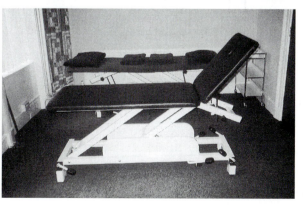

c.

The Treatment Table

The massage table is also known variously as the 'couch' or 'plinth' and the three terms are used inter-changeably.

Students and newly qualified practitioners usually acquire wooden framed portable massage tables. The meaurements of the couch are usually in the following range: 1.9 metres long by 70 cms wide and between 56–66 cms high. Manufacturers offer variations on these measurements to suit individuals. They represent good value for money, are a good stand-by even when the therapist eventually purchases a more expensive model, they are easily portable for home visits or outside sporting events and they have an excellent second-hand value.

There are heavier, more solid, fixed height wooden treatment tables that are permanent fixtures within the clinic. These are more expensive than portable tables but will last a therapist for many years and, possibly, until retirement!

The more popular types, though, are the electrical and hydraulic plinths that are easily adjustable. Electric tables have several disadvantages over the hydraulic tables and the electrical components must be checked by an approved electrical engineer annually to meet Health and Safety regulations and insurance criteria.

I would recommend that new practitioners save a portion of every fee until they can afford a good foot-pump actioned hydraulic adjustable plinth. Many retailers will bargain with you in what is a competitive field. Second-hand hydraulic plinths may have a problem with the hydraulic mechanism – the most expensive component of the table. So check out second-hand plinths carefully before purchasing.

Hydraulic and electrically operated plinths make life so much easier for the patients and for the therapist, too. These plinths can be adjusted to enable easier mounting and dismounting for the patient and also adjust to the most suitable working height for the therapist. This helps ward off some of the stresses and strains that develop when working seven or eight hours a day at a fixed height table.

The profession of remedial massage is quite tough physically and some therapists develop painful conditions of the hands, elbows, shoulders and spine that are attributable to their work and especially to fixed height couches. The therapist, thus, becomes a patient.

The treatment table should be covered by a large towel or a purpose-made couch cover. These are readily available in various colours and sizes from specialist outlets.

Pillows are also used to support the head and the legs. When the patient is lying prone (face down) they usually require three pillows. One to support the feet to prevent friction on the toes and possible cramping of the muscles of the sole of the foot, a second pillow to support the abdomen and the third pillow to support the head and shoulders. When the patient is treated in the supine (face up) position, two pillows are used, one to support the head and the other to support the knees. The purpose of these pillows is to enable the patient to relax all the muscles of the body and to get the patient to relax as fully as possible.

The Use of Towels

Once the patient has removed the clothing as directed by the therapist to enable the therapist to examine and treat, the patient should be provided with a towel to cover themselves until the examination or treatment commences.

A patient who requires an examination or treatment to the back will be required to undress down to their underwear. The towel is provided so that the patient does not have to stand or walk about with so few clothes on. When the time comes for the examination or the treatment, the part of the body, in this case the back, can be uncovered quite quickly.

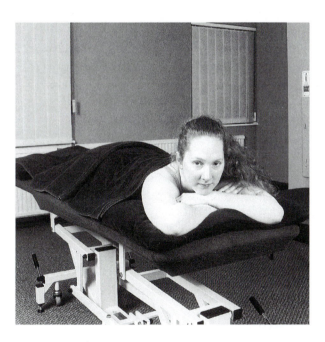

◄ *Figure 20*
Towelled and relaxed awaiting treatment.

Once on the plinth, the patient is covered by two large towels. One towel is doubled with the open end at the feet; the other is doubled with the open end at the neck. This will bring the two folds at the centre into such a position that there is no possible chance of the body being exposed due to the overlapping of both towels across the centre of the body.

When treating the shoulder, a portion of the upper towel is turned back, thus exposing the part of the body which is under treatment and keeping the rest of the body well covered. After treating the shoulder area they are then covered by the towel and the next part of the body requiring treatment is uncovered.

Correct use of the towels is one of the characteristics of a well-trained therapist. Correct use of the towels makes the patient feel safe and secure, keeps the patient warm and helps the patient to feel at ease and relaxed.

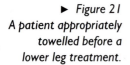
▶ *Figure 21*
A patient appropriately towelled before a lower leg treatment.

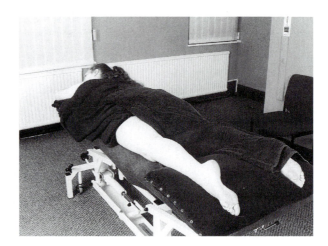

As the patient begins to relax on the treatment table, blood pressure lowers and the circulation pattern changes and with these changes the body begins to feel cooler. The folded towels in a well heated room prevent this feeling of cooling-off. Correct use of the towels is essential for good and professional massage treatment. It will tell the patient much about the therapist and anything less than correct use of towels should not be tolerated.

There is also a correct procedure for turning a patient from prone to supine positions on the plinth. Firstly, check that there is no equipment near to the plinth that will impede the movement.

The therapist removes the pillow from under the patient's abdomen and opens the upper towel to its full length so that it completely covers the patient. The therapist then places one hand in the centre of the patient's back to prevent the opened towel from slipping. The folded lower towel is now removed with the other hand.

The single covering towel is held firmly by both hands and the patient is requested to turn on to his back towards the therapist. Thus, there will be no exposure of the patient's body because the towel will not slip during the turning action. Double the two towels as before and place a pillow under the patient's knees so that the abdominal muscles are completely relaxed and the patient is ready for further treatment.

Oils and Creams

The principal function of the massage medium is to reduce friction between the therapist's hands and the patient's body and thus allow the massage movements to flow smoothly. Some types of massage may be done without lubricant but it is generally accepted that some medium is required. There is a variety of oils and creams available as well as the more specialised essential oils of the aromatherapist.

Powder

Powder as a massage medium is frequently referred to in books but I do not personally know a therapist who uses powder as a regular massage medium. It is worth noting that Tod (1951) claimed that powder was the most common lubricant used in massage; the finest French chalk, starch powder or mixtures of starch, boracic and chalk or zinc may be used. It is not particularly good at reducing friction, creates a mess in the treatment room and usually leads to a sustained bout of sneezing by both patient and therapist.

Oils

The use of oils is traditional in massage therapy and most are based on nut and seed oils. They provide a good lubrication provided they are not over-applied but oils have a tendency to stain linen and clothing. Do not try and store them for too long as they will deteriorate and become rancid. Mineral oils have the taint of carginogen, have no nutritional value and tend to block the pores of the skin.

Essential oils are concentrated essences of plants. There are contra-indications to the use of some otherwise popular oils, for example, the use of clary sage in pregnancy and also it is not a good idea if either the recipient or the therapist has to drive afterwards. If the therapist wishes to use essential oils, it is the responsibility of the therapist to gain some training and qualification in the use of these powerful oils before using them on their patients.

I would admit to the use of lavender oil and tea tree oil on a regular basis but for self-treatment rather than using them on my patients.

Creams

Creams are more manageable than oils and provide good lubrication and little mess especially so in that creams tend not to stain clothing and linen.

All lubricants should be stored at room temperature in closed containers. Pump action containers are preferred for ease of handling and safer risk from contamination.

Some patients may have an allergic reaction to a certain massage medium. I can remember that I, a therapist, had a reaction to a certain brand of massage lotion some years ago. Nuts provoke strong reactions in some people and a nut oil used for treatment may also provoke a reaction. Some patients have sensitive skin and may react to one product but not to another. A good idea would be the purchase of a hypoallergenic lubricant, i.e. one that the manufacturers assure you has undergone lengthy testing and did not cause any allergic reactions on the subjects used in the tests. This could be used on patients with a history of reactions to other lubricants.

The most frequent problem with the massage medium is that students and newly qualified practitioners use far too much and their massage treatment is slippery. However, with a little experience most therapists find that they quickly determine how much, or indeed, how little of a certain lubricant to use on each individual.

Examination of the Patient

Treatment should not begin until the patient has been examined by the therapist. This 'golden rule', referred to by Cassar (1999), must always be followed and to treat a patient without carrying out a thorough examination would be most unprofessional.

Every new patient must be fully and thoroughly examined. After the examination process has been completed, the therapist should be in a position to decide if there are any contra-indications to massage treatment, to assess the patient's problems and to formulate and discuss with the patient a plan of treatment for that patient's condition. To begin treatment without an examination may be dangerous to the patient and, if not dangerous, it is unlikely that the treatment will be beneficial to the patient.

The art of examination is crucial to the success of the therapist's treatment. It is not an easy art to acquire and the therapist needs to be well instructed during training and then to work hard at the various skills required when in practice.

The examination process begins the moment the therapist first comes into contact with the patient. It is the start of a very special relationship between the patient and the therapist and this is further reason for the therapist to have as professionally expert an examination procedure as possible. Patients should be made aware of the confidentiality of this relationship and should feel secure in the knowledge that whatever is said or done will remain a matter solely between therapist and patient, unless they give permission for the therapist to divulge any of the information.

Many thousands of years ago, Hippocrates wrote about the vital importance of relaxation in the process of healing and that healing only commences once the patient relaxes. Mostly, patients come to the therapist because they are in pain. They are probably anxious and, especially if new to massage and manipulation, ill-at-ease as well. *"... all professions are a conspiracy against the laity,"* quoted by Mitchell and Cormack (1998) from George Bernard Shaw. An expert, caring examination of the patient, should help bring about a relaxation in the patient and allow the healing process to begin. The opposite, unfortunately, is also true!

Procedure for Examination

The procedure for examining a patient has evolved over many years. It was a pleasure to read the invaluable book specifically about examination procedures by Apley and Solomon (1997) in which the authors outlined a simple and effective method of examination. This procedure to be followed in the examination of patients is summed up by the words: **"LISTEN – LOOK – FEEL – MOVE."**

Listen to the Patient

The therapist should listen to their patients at all times and not only during the examination process.

The new patient coming to your treatment room will probably be in some physical discomfort and will also be rather anxious and apprehensive about their condition and your method of treatment. By putting the patient at ease and giving him or her the opportunity to tell a sympathetic professional about the injury or condition triggers the healing process. Listening and talking to patients elicits information but it also has a therapeutic quality. It can be the start of healing; the patient relaxes and begins to feel better.

Patients want and need to tell you about their condition. Reflect for a moment and think about situations from your own experience when you have gone to a medical professional with a problem and found yourself in and out of the consultation room in double quick time with a prescription in your hand and a feeling of frustration. You have not had the opportunity to talk nor to be listened to.

It may only require an encouraging smile and a simple question or statement from you to the patient to set the process in motion. For example:

"You have made an appointment with me about your backache, Mr. Smith. Tell me about it........"

"Good morning Mrs. Jones, I believe you've got a painful shoulder. When did the pain start?"

The therapist needs to ask the right questions to enable the patient to talk, to give their account of their injury or condition. And then the therapist must listen carefully to the patient. The therapist needs to find out from the patient the following information:

1.   The onset of the condition. When did the discomfort begin?
     When did it start to hurt?
2.   The site of pain. Where does it hurt?
3.   Has the patient had this condition before, for example back pain?
4.   Is it any better or does it become worse at certain times of the day?
5.   Has the patient taken any medication and what effect did it have?
6.   Has the patient seen his or her doctor or had any other treatment
     in connection with the presenting condition?
7.   Does it affect the patient's sleep patterns?
8.   How does it affect work, leisure activities, everyday living?
9.   What are their work and leisure activities?
10. Lifestyle in general, e.g. diet, alcohol, tobacco.
11. Is the patient currently being treated for any other medical conditions?
12. History of patient's previous illnesses, accidents, in fact a
     comprehensive medical history.

What other information, apart from the medical, can the therapist glean from this conversation with the patient? Some aspects of the patient's personality, attitudes and characteristics may become apparent during the conversation and may assist the therapist in making an assessment of a particular patient.

This part of the examination process, often called taking the patient's history, must be done in a relaxed and unhurried manner. The patient should feel at ease and be given time to think, answer and discuss. Allow plenty of time for this and do not be in such a hurry to commence treatment. A colleague, an orthopaedic surgeon, in conversation informed me that he expects to devote a period of twenty minutes plus to listening to a new patient and taking the patient's history before proceeding to the rest of the examination. My own clinical experiences would fully support this statement.

I much prefer not to make notes whilst listening to a patient. Nor do I use a tape recorder. Many patients view note-taking as an intrusion, a disruption of the process and their answers tend to become briefer, vaguer and less spontaneous. Trying to make a note of everything a patient says usually means that the therapist misses out on vital information because of the distraction imposed by the very process of making the notes. Notes can be made later, perhaps whilst the patient undresses for the next part of the examination or immediately after the first session is completed.

Most patients feel uncomfortable to a greater or lesser degree, when faced with the prospect of speaking into a tape recorder. I want the patient to feel able to relax and I try to remove anything that interferes with this.

Patients must be assured and feel confident that whatever is said or discussed will remain confidential. All information exchanged between patient and therapist is confidential and should remain so. None of the information should ever be divulged to a third person without the patient's written permission, for example, information about the patient supplied to a solicitor in regard to a legal action. There may be other instances in which the therapist feels that the bond of confidentiality may need to be broken and it may be that the therapist should take advice from his professional body or from the patient's medical practitioner.

Otherwise, confidentiality should be strictly observed. Patients must be able to feel secure in the knowledge that you will not discuss them or their conditions with any other person. Similarly, if a patient in your treatment room wishes to discuss another patient, then conversation must be quickly steered away from the subject and the patient be firmly but politely informed that this type of discussion just does not take place in your treatment room.

It is, of course, most important that the therapist does keep a record of the examination and, later, of treatments. Again, the failure to keep records is most unprofessional and may lead to serious consequences at a later date. Records must be kept in a safe and secure place where they cannot be looked at or taken by a third party.

Look – Visual Examination of the Patient

The therapist should use the sense of sight in a constructive, diagnostic way. Look and see. Take in as much information about the patient from the very first sighting. To quote Hoppenfeld (1976): *"Inspection begins as the patient enters the examination room."* First impressions about the patient should not be ignored and will give the therapist valuable information about the patient.

Evaluate the balance and symmetry of the patient as the patient stands and walks. Look for unevenness and distorted movement as the patient may try to compensate for what should be smooth normal movement. Andry (in Keith, 1919) observed that corpulent men and pregnant women walked with a straight back even an overextended one, because they were overloaded in front. A youth who stooped was prescribed for by visual examination alone – the natural way to bring the muscles of the spine into action and give him an erect carriage was to make him carry a burden in the front of his body or hang a weight upon his breast.

During my time in practice, I was a fairly frequent visitor to many of the excellent local restaurants and part of my evening was often spent watching the restaurant staff as they moved about the establishment. I was, on many occasions, able to say to a waiter or waitress at the end of the evening, "How long have you suffered with your back?" or hip or knee. They usually answered, with some astonishment, that they had a long-standing problem that was of increasing concern. I always made sure I had some business cards with me on these occasions and, over the years, built up a good patient base from the catering industry simply by using my eyes.

The visual examination of patients is an important part of the examination process. It is partly informal as in watching how a patient walks or sits down or removes a coat. Much information can be gained from observing the patient's gait and their sitting and standing posture.

The visual examination can also be more formal. After listening to the patient's history, the therapist may then ask the patient to remove some of their clothing in order to carry out this more formal visual examination. I rarely actually said to a patient, "Stand there I want to examine you." So many, upon hearing these words, instantly assume a completely uncharacteristic pose; they stand how they think I want them to stand; like parade ground soldiers.

A visual examination may be done quite quickly at this stage. The therapist looks for the obvious; for anything out of the ordinary and for a picture of balance and symmetry. Having got the general picture, the patient may be positioned on the treatment table for closer local scrutiny. The type of conditions to be looked for in a general visual examination would include; scoliosis, exaggerated lordosis or kyphosis, tight muscles, atrophied muscles, over-developed muscles that may have been caused by repetitive overuse, knee or foot abnormalities. Do not underestimate a patient's feet; a good podiatrist will always be willing to tell you how many back conditions, headaches even, are caused by a 'fallen' arch.

Apley and Solomon advised that the therapist does not touch the patient during the visual examination. Once touch is engaged the visual information is switched off.

Feel – Examination of the Patient by Palpation

Touch is one of the primary senses. The skilled therapist uses touch to investigate, to explore and thus gain information or supplement information already gained by other means such as sight. Field (1997) discussed this at some length in his definitive book about palpation and added other qualities such as searching, tracking or tracing out, to examine systematically in detail by feeling. Thus, palpation is more than just the use of the hands to feel the patient; it is to feel and investigate systematically.

Palpation appears to be a combination of touch, feel, examination, sensory feedback and interpretation through previous experience. The skills are used in a methodical way to enable specific information about the patient to be acquired.

Sanderson (1998) stated that experience gives the massage therapist the ability to distinguish between the various kinds of tissue according to how they feel. The significance of this statement is that the art of touching and feeling a patient's tissues (palpation) is not one that comes to the therapist purely as a gift. It is an art that is acquired over a period of time by dint of constant practise. It must be learned, practised and developed with conscious effort from the first day as a student and right through the long years of the career of the practitioner.

The patient quickly becomes aware of the skill and ability of the person performing the examination and reacts accordingly. A skilled therapist opens a two-way communication between patient and practitioner and information is forthcoming. The patient feels at ease and relaxed...again, the opposite is also true!

The examination must be undertaken with care and sensitivity, precision and gentleness for the patient to become confident and relaxed. The patient then will begin to relay information, some of it verbal and some of it non-verbal, back to the therapist. The therapist should pay attention to the facial expressions and body language of the patient. Occasionally, body language is a more reliable indicator than the patient's spoken answer. The therapist may palpate a certain area of tissue and ask the patient if they felt pain. The patient may reply, "No," but at the same time the therapist notices a facial grimace or white knuckles gripping the edge of the examination table.

The process of examination by palpation does not cease at the conclusion of the examination. Rather, palpation will continue during treatment for, as muscles relax and joints ease as a result of massage, the therapist will be able to palpate even more deeply into the tissues undergoing the remedial treatment and be able to add to the information already gained.

Move – Examination of the Patient by Movement

The next phase of the examination is to examine the patient by movement. That is to use active and passive movements of the areas about which the patient has told the therapist, in which pain, stiffness or restriction of movement is occurring.

The therapist explains to the patient exactly what movements are required and then demonstrates the movement to the patient.

The patient is then asked to perform the movements by himself, by using his own muscles to try to complete the required range of movement. Ask the patient, where appropriate, to perform the movement with the uninjured side, followed by movement of the injured part. This will give the therapist an example of normal movement with which to compare the range of movement of the injured limb.

For example, a patient complaining of pain and restriction around the right shoulder, is asked to perform the range of movements normally possible at the joint, firstly by using the left shoulder and then by using the right or injured shoulder. This is examination by active movement and the therapist will be able to assess the range of movements at both shoulders and compare one side with the other.

In passive movement testing, the therapist moves the patient's body parts through the range of movement for him. The patient may not be able to perform the full range of active movements. Passive testing serves to eliminate the patient's muscle function from consideration and the probable cause of the problem and indicate an injury involving the actual joint structures.

When carrying out an examination by movement the patient should be as relaxed as possible. If the patient is apprehensive his muscles will become tense and the examiner will not be able to get a true picture. The passive movements should be performed smoothly and gently and with support, to afford the joint the opportunity to show any restriction or pain.

Contra-indications to Treatment by Massage

During the examination procedure, the therapist must be aware that not every person who presents for massage treatment will benefit from the treatment. In some cases there will not only be lack of benefit from the treatment but the patient may be seriously harmed and possibly suffer fatal consequences from an inappropriate treatment.

There are a number of contra-indications to massage of which every therapist should be aware at all times. It is the duty and obligation of the therapist to rule out the presence of any conditions in which massage may have detrimental effects (Salvo, 1999).

Conditions in which massage may be harmful to the patient may be termed absolute contra-indications, i.e. no massage treatment whatsoever. An example of an absolute contra-indication to massage is pyrexia or fever. Massage treatment of such a patient runs the risk of increasing the infection by stimulating the circulation. Usually, contra-indications are taken to mean no massage treatments to certain, affected parts of the body. Many conditions may have partial or relative contra-indications where the therapist must exercise caution.

Massage may be administered in these cases but care must be taken to ensure the patient is safe and comfortable. The following is a list of conditions that may contra-indicate massage to the specific area of injury or lesion but may be beneficial in reducing anxiety and stress or be valuable therapeutically in areas of the body distant to the area where the condition is located:

1. Infectious (and other) skin conditions and abnormalities, e.g. rashes, impetigo, ringworm, scabies, severe itching and any fungal or bacterial infection.
2. Do not massage over any area containing a foreign object, for example, a splinter, glass, metal. Massage may cause further damage to the tissues and there is a chance of infection to both therapist and patient.
3. Varicose veins (see vascular conditions).
4. Pregnancy, especially during the first three months.
5. Acute inflammation.
6. Recent wounds, recent surgery, cuts, abrasions, haematomas, bruising. Allow reasonable healing time or there is risk of further damage to the injured tissues. After surgery, e.g. appendicitis, get the approval of the patient's physician or GP.
7. Cancer patients; massage is often strongly designated as a contra-indication but, please read, *"Medicine Hands"* by Gayle MacDonald for a thoroughly

expert and professional view on this contentious issue. There is a significant part that massage treatments can play on patients with this condition.

8. Rheumatoid Arthritis and other inflammatory illnesses like Systemic Lupus Erythematosus, Crohn's Disease. Each condition and each patient requires careful examination and planning and therapists should establish liaison with patient's medical practitioner.

9. Infectious diseases, for example, 'flu, measles, mumps. Do not treat by massage during the period of infection and, again check with the patient's GP.

10. Chronic constipation; the patient must be referred for further medical examination.

11. Frequent headaches; these patients should be referred to their medical practitioner.

12. Diabetes; therapists must check with the patient's GP before treatments commence because of other medical implications. My experience with diabetic patients was that circulation, especially of the extremities, was helped.

13. Severe or intractable pain especially of sudden onset and, in my clinical experience, with middle-aged to elderly patients. Once or perhaps twice each year, a middle-aged patient with sudden onset severe pain in the thoracic or cervical spine/occipital areas was encountered. Light and relaxing effleurage tended to make the patients feel worse rather than easing the pain. My procedure for these patients was to contact the patient's GP practice by phone and request an early appointment for the patient. Following up the patient later generally discovered that the patient was suffering from a tumour.

14. Hepatitis.

15. Umbilical hernias.

16. Toxaemia.

17. Patients with allergies for which they are receiving medical attention.

18. Any person who will not disclose their medical history.

19. A person under the influence of alcohol or other substances, even legitimate medication that inhibit the patient's response or ability to give feedback regarding discomfort or pain.

20. Psychological/mental health; again each case must be judged by the therapist and medical and psychological advice and opinion sought before treating. As there are conditions where massage treatment could be very beneficial there are also other conditions which may be aggravated simply by touching the patient.

21. Anything of which the therapist is unsure, e.g. a patient with an already diagnosed kidney problem, a heart condition and receiving treatment.

If there are doubts about anything, further checks should be done with the patient and with the patient's physician before massage treatment starts.

Assessment and Planning

Upon completion of the examination procedure, the therapist should be in a position to complete the assessment of the patient, to be able to tell the patient about his findings from the examination and discuss these with the patient.

For example, based upon the patient's description of the incidents leading up to the injury, the location of the pain pointed out by the patient, the therapist's visual and palpatory examinations and the results of testing by movement, the therapist may be able to say to the patient that the injury is one to the hamstring group of muscles or muscles around the shoulder joint or the ligaments of the knee joint. Most patients want to know the nature of their injury. "What is it?" is usually followed quickly by "When will it be better?" or "When can I start training?"

Explain to the patient the nature of their condition and how your treatment plan will help their condition or injury. Each patient has his or her individual problem or condition. The patient may be in pain and is probably feeling unwell or fearful and, in this state it is important that not only do you positively and actively care for your patients but that your patients know that you care for them. This is the foundation upon which your remedial massage treatments are based.

The sometimes, impersonal approach of orthodox medicine, or the dehumanisation of orthodox medicine described by Reilly (1998) stemmed in part from the delusion that technology had made caring redundant. What did it matter who gave you your prescription so long as it was effective? In the clinical situation the personal touch is present and this personal interest is what the patient expects from the remedial therapist.

The next step in dealing with the patient is to discuss their personal and individual treatment plan. After a concise explanation of the injury or condition, the therapist will then discuss in detail with the patient how he will treat the patient's condition; to discuss, explain and agree with the patient on the approximate number of treatments and the frequency of treatments.

Of course, the patient must be told about the contents of the treatment sessions, about the different massage techniques and their effects, any movements or mobilisations and why they are performed. Possibly the therapist may include electrotherapy in the treatments and this should be explained to the patient in advance. Inform the patient about any 'homework' that may be included in the treatment plan, i.e. a simple exercise routine in which the patient will perform mobilising movements and/or stretches on a daily basis before the next appointment.

Each patient should be regarded as an active participant in their treatment. Without their positive help, the treatments given will not be effective and beneficial. The patient who becomes actively and positively involved in his or her treatment will respond more positively and more quickly than the patient who is apathetic and negative or the patient who demands that the therapist 'cures' them and, often, in a single session.

The whole approach, the ambience of the remedial massage treatment room should make it easier for therapists to adopt what Mitchell and McCormack (1998) described as a 'more collaborative style' with their patients.

The remedial massage therapist treats by massage techniques, mobilising of joints and 'stretching' muscles and by basic exercise movements, some of which the patient may also perform at home. The therapist may also have 'other strings to his bow' (Duncombe, 1970), for example, a knowledge and mastery of neuromuscular massage techniques, manipulative skills, perhaps some training in electrotherapy, lymphatic drainage or thermal therapy. From this menu of treatments, the therapist will extract what he feels each individual patient requires and create a plan designed to treat each patient according to the needs of that individual patient.

Advertising Your Practice

The question of advertising taxes many therapists. Does one pay for adverts in national or local papers? What about magazines? For the therapist most advertising in newspapers and magazines is a waste of money, unless the therapist has really done some homework and is sure of reaching a target population.

Do not be seduced by the many offers that come along. Especially beware of telephone salespersons who will tell you that they have a marvellous nationwide offer at half price due to an unexpected cancellation. However you must book with them now because today is the deadline for sending the copy off to the printer. It's all so easy, just give your credit card number. Do not fall for this one. The chances are that you are being conned. Do not buy anything over the phone from people you do not know very well.

Similarly, beware of the compilers of registers and directories, often bogus, who want to take your money over the phone. Another variation on this theme is the man who rings up speaking on behalf of the local police station or the fire service or underprivileged children. That is the impression he seeks to give when, in fact, he is seeking your advertisement in a publication that has little to do with the police or any other cause mentioned. If the offer is of interest request copies of previous publications or get in touch with the charity mentioned before committing yourself to paying.

Most patients live within a couple of miles radius of your clinic. If you advertise, target this population. I took advice from my tutors and mentors and I found that very localised advertising paid the best dividends. For example, the local church's newsletter or the village fête brochure. Not only is the advertising rate a low one, the publication will be looked at by local people and you are also seen to be supporting local events and activities.

If you decide to take out a modest advert in the local newspaper, do so for a series of six weekly insertions. A one-off advertisement will be missed by most of the potential clients but a series of six will have some impact, especially by the time the fourth or fifth advertisement appears. It is at this time that the telephone should begin to ring with prospective patients. The chances are that the local newspaper will do a deal with you and give you not only a reduced rate but also some editorial coverage.

However, the best advertising for any practitioner is by patients who appreciate the treatments you have given them. Every patient you treat is entitled to the best possible treatment – the best possible care and attention. The patient should go away from your treatment room ready to recommend you to family and friends. This is in fact what happens.

As a student, I was told that if I treated to the best of my ability I would not have to advertise. My patients would advertise on my behalf; word of mouth recommendation is the best recommendation and the best way of advertising.

I would like to introduce you to some of my patients, ones whom I termed 'pivotal patients' because of the positive effects they had on the development of my practice. These were the patients whose word of mouth recommendations helped me through the early days in practice and made it possible for my practice to grow and become successful.

Pivotal Patients

Mary

Mary was a middle aged, gregarious lady who worked in the local shop. She came to see me some twelve months after I had moved into the area and opened my clinic. I was aware that all my patients were 'in-comers', people who had moved to the area like myself, and commuted to the nearby towns to work. I had not treated any of the 'native' population so far.

Mary complained to all and sundry and, on this occasion to me, of a 'frozen shoulder' although she demonstrated quite actively that it was not 'frozen'. Rather her shoulder was limited in certain movements, in abduction and lateral rotation and the movements hurt her when she had to reach behind her in the shop to take items down from shelves. She informed me that medical opinion considered that it would be, 'two years of a job'.

I treated Mary by neck and shoulder massage and the standard mobilising techniques for the shoulder. After three treatments she was re-tested and by her own declaration she had recovered the full range of movements in the injured shoulder. She could move freely and without pain.

What I did not know was that Mary's shoulder was the subject of an on-going debate in the shop; a real life medical 'soap'. Mary's treatments now assumed the leading role and her sessions with me were reported on and debated at length with a succession of regular shoppers.

Soon after Mary recovered the full use of her shoulder, my telephone became much busier as people started to make appointments for massage treatments. I had passed my test as far as the locals were concerned by the successful treatment of Mary's shoulder.

Mrs. H

One February evening in the early 1980's, accompanied by lashing rain and sixty mile an hour gales, I kept an appointment at a local church hall to speak to a ladies group – all five of them on this occasion.

I wondered for a moment what on earth I was doing even coming out of the house on such a dreadful night to speak to such a small audience. I gave my talk about massage and demonstrated some basic techniques on my wife who had thoughtfully accompanied me. A few gentle questions from the ladies and then an invitation to pick the winning ticket for that evening's draw. I gave out five business cards and received a pot of homemade marmalade for my wages. A less than satisfactory evening?

Some years later during a day of enforced inactivity brought about by a snow storm that had patients cancelling appointments left, right and centre, I decided to check through the patient files. The objective was to find how many referrals had come from a certain Mrs. H, one of the 'Five' from that awful February evening.

It took almost the complete day to follow-up the referrals (which are marked on each patients' card) and add up the number of appointments and the fees. At the end of the process, I traced referrals from Mrs. H to so many patients that, in a period of just under five years, these referrals accounted for almost twenty thousand pounds in fees. All of this from one lady who had been impressed by our talk and demonstration. She referred her husband and her children, her relatives and her friends and they in turn referred others to me for treatment.

Mrs. H never came for treatment for herself until one day many years later. Her son phoned unbeknown to her, to ask me to call at the farm to treat her sprained ankle on which she had been hobbling around for some days. It was the first time I met her since the talk in the church hall. On this occasion I waived my fee.

Mrs. B

Mrs. B came to my treatment room one morning and, although she lived only a few doors away, I had not seen her before in my professional capacity. She sounded desperate and a touch angry as she told me her story. She had arthritis of the right knee, the result of a motorcycle accident some thirty years previously.

Her knee was deformed, the muscles atrophied, the joint appeared to be fixed in flexion and she had to wear a very noticeably built-up boot on the right foot. She walked slowly with the aid of a stick. Her treatment over the years had been one of taking painkillers and an emphasis on rest from any activity that might aggravate the condition.

Now at the age of sixty she had had enough of being an invalid and wanted to get out and about like a normal person – to summarise her own words. Could I help with massage? I asked her what she wanted out of my treatments; what would be our goals. She listed them as follows:

- "To get rid of the 'cripple' boot."
- "To throw away the walking stick."
- "To walk normally in normal shoes."

Looking through my treatment room window, she pointed to a nearby hill saying:

- "I want to walk up there again!"

I treated her twice each week and used the basic massage techniques, except for tapotement at this stage, on the whole of her affected leg. I used passive movements for her foot, ankle, knee and hip.

We began gentle stretching exercises especially for the hamstrings which were both atrophied and hypertonic. I employed a little faradic muscle stimulation to the quadriceps during the first few treatments. Mrs. B did some gentle stretching of her hamstrings and then we started some easy strengthening exercises. We began the strengthening exercises on the quadriceps and did sets (three sets of eight repetitions) of leg extension exercises with an oven glove draped over her ankle and a small tin of beans in each compartment.

I made an appointment for her to see some colleagues at the local college. They worked a minor miracle for her and quickly provided an insert for a normal shoe that could also be transferred to other shoes. At last, the repugnant boot was thrown into the dustbin and Mrs. B could wear ordinary shoes like normal people.

Needless to say, she progressed very quickly and within six months she had regained almost full extension of her leg. The muscles had flourished with massage, movement, stretching and exercise and the deformed knee was not so obvious any more as it was surrounded by healthy muscle tissue.

She fulfilled the requirement exactly that in the application of massage and exercise there is one condition that is absolutely essential for success; the patient must be an active, not a passive agent in the treatment. Ling is reported as stating that the main agent in recovery was the patient's will to recover. There is no miracle in healing except that which is brought about by hard work – hard thinking by the therapist followed by hard effort by the patient. Deane (1918) wrote that any method of treatment that lacks the essential factors of stimulating and encouraging man's own power of will-to-do stands condemned.

The walking stick went the way of the boot and Mrs. B became a regular figure walking around the neighbourhood and, at about this time, she called in to inform me that she had walked up the hill with her husband and achieved the last of her stated goals.

For years, family and friends had been used to this lady, crippled by arthritis, walking with the aid of a stick and built-up boot. All of a sudden there is a transformation and everybody wanted to know all about it. Mrs. B's treatments and the progress she made had a big impact on my growing practice.

Once the treatments started and with encouragement, Mrs. B did most of the work with a little bit of help from me and my colleagues. We did not cure her arthritis and some days she reported that it was still as painful. What we achieved between us was a more positive way for her to cope with the problems of her arthritic knee and to lead a fuller and more active life.

Mr. P

A man telephoned for an appointment and told me that he was severely affected by diabetes. He informed me that he had eye problems and problems with his circulation. To walk for more than fifty yards left him in pain and fatigued. Would regular massage help his circulation?

He came for his first appointment and I conducted an in-depth examination and discovered that he had several more medical problems including hypertension and a long-standing cardiac condition. His main concern, however, seemed to be focused on his problem with his circulation. We both decided that it would be dangerous to plunge straight into massage treatments and he gave me permission to approach his GP.

The doctor gave his approval for foot and leg massage and the treatment sessions started with effleurage and petrissage of the leg and a foot massage. I was instructed by the GP to look out for any cuts, bruises or infection around the foot and ankle and to report any such wound to the practice nurse immediately.

My patient was a very respected self-made businessman with some forty years business experience in my locality. He responded well to the treatments and progress was measured by how far he could walk before he felt the need to sit down for a rest.

I also found out that he was a season ticket holder at the local soccer club and that there had been concern expressed by officials at the ground about his fitness to actually attend matches. This, then, was the motivation to come for treatments. Or so I thought....

After eight weeks, we sat down and had a discussion about progress and he informed me that he could walk for a good fifteen minutes before he needed to rest – progress of about twelve minutes from the start of treatment. I was quite pleased at this until he asked me could I treat his impotence, a side-effect of diabetes.

This was a new problem for me and, after discussion with colleagues and some hurried reading, we decided to try several of the acupressure points from a book supplied by a colleague. Once started, he self-administered the acupressure techniques whilst I continued with the remedial massage.

It worked, too. Some three weeks afterwards he came in for his remedial massage treatment and found some difficulty in keeping the smile off his face. His impotence had been defeated. He attributed much of the credit to my treatments and recommended me to his many friends and acquaintances.

Mrs. HA

Mrs. HA had her appointment made on her behalf by her husband who sounded curt and brusque and emphasised that I was his last hope rather than hers.

The patient reported continuing headaches over an eighteen-year period. They started at the same time as she was studying for her A-Levels and had been a dominating feature of her life during professional accountancy training, early career, marriage and from then on up to the present.

She had been examined by her own doctor and several consultants at various hospitals in the area. X-ray investigation to the cervical spine had been unhelpful and had not shown any cause for the head pain. She had also undergone brain scans on two occasions. Both were negative but I tried to imagine the fear and apprehension that she had suffered whilst awaiting both the scans and the outcome on each occasion. She told me that she was still half convinced she had some very obscure form of tumour that the investigations had missed. There were no other contra-indications to massage treatments.

The patient had all the signs and symptoms that accompany chronic and prolonged pain. These included loss of concentration, chronic feeling of fatigue, irritability with everyone and a sense of isolation and loss of relationships and contact with family and friends (presumably why the husband expressed concern in his own way when making the initial appointment).

She appeared to be suffering from a categorisation of headache noted by Edeling (1988) as somewhat controversial. Because objective tests failed to show any pathology and stress-related muscle contraction of the neck and head muscles seemed to be the only significant findings, this common, non-vascular chronic headache has become known as a 'tension' headache.

Edeling quoted from the *Journal of the American Medical Association* (1962) a report that effectively stated that sustained muscle contraction of the head and neck muscles was the primary cause of this type of headache and had put forward the term 'muscle contraction headache'. Because of some contradictions in subsequent research the terminology was changed to 'chronic daily headache.' Chronic tension headache was considered a difficult therapeutic problem by Kunkel (1991).

No one had found a cause for her headaches nor had anyone found a cure and she survived on a diet of rest in darkened rooms and painkillers – and she still worked full-time and looked after her husband and children. She looked pained and in pain, desperate and anxious.

The treatment plan was quite straightforward; neck and shoulder massage in a calm and quiet environment and a programme of daily neck mobilising exercises. I had found with many patients suffering from headaches that massage, mobilisation techniques and neck traction was quite effective and Edeling, in her interesting book, recommended the effectiveness of a range of physical treatments similar to those used for this particular patient.

The patient was massaged firstly in the prone position and then in supine position with particular attention to the muscles linking head and spine and shoulders (see Neck and Shoulder Massage, pp.111–135). I employed the following remedial massage sequence; effleurage, frictions, petrissage. After the massage I performed a series of passive movements that took the joints of the neck through their full range of movements and tractions.

Mrs. HA remained completely silent during her initial treatment and left with hardly a word. The second and third treatments were conducted in exactly the same manner with any questions answered by her with simple positives or negatives. She was scheduled for two treatments a week for three weeks with a review at the end of the six sessions.

The patient underwent a marked change between treatment three and treatment four. She smiled as she came into the room and asked how I was. There was a startling change in her manner, her bearing and posture, her attitude and even in her choice of clothing which had previously been dark and sombre and now contained bright red and yellow. What she reported to me was of more significance.

She began to feel relaxed during the first treatment and felt that a lot of tightness had gone from her neck and from around her head during the treatment. The mobilising movements allowed her to realise that she could in fact move her head freely and that it was not restricted. The traction movements felt to her as if they were lifting great weights from around her neck and head.

Most importantly, she said that she had been free of headaches since the second treatment and had taken no medication since the third treatment. She had been a little hesitant to admit to herself, let alone to me or to anyone else that she no longer had the head pains, but it was true. The truth took a little time to overcome the apprehension that the pain would quickly return. She said that she could see more clearly and that everything looked brighter and more precisely defined. She was sure now that the eighteen years of pain had ended.

She completed the course of treatments and remained free of pain. After the review she was discharged with the proviso that if the headaches even hinted of a return she would telephone for immediate treatment.

Not all headache patients respond so dramatically and each patient must be examined with care and referred to their doctor if any of the symptoms give the therapist any cause for concern. However, headaches of the type displayed by this patient are quite common and are also responsive to remedial massage treatment.

I did not see her for two years but occasionally friends she recommended came to me for treatment and talked about the marvellous changes that had occurred in her life after years of problems. It was then only by accident that I met her in the town centre. I greeted her and though her reply was bright I got the impression she did not recognise me. I reminded her who I was and referred to her treatment. She replied: "Do you know, I'd forgotten I ever had the headaches. I wonder, was it really me?"

She told me that, among other things, she had changed her job just as she finished the treatments and everything else seemed to improve coincidentally with the treatments. I could only guess at what had happened in her life but we were both sure that the massage treatments set the changes in motion.

Working With Doctors

Everyone treated by a remedial massage therapist is, in all likelihood, on the patient list of a GP. The local GPs find out about the activities of a remedial massage therapist very quickly from their patients. The GP is often aware of any new complementary or alternative therapist in his area long before the therapist suspects his or her activities are known about.

After discussion with several GPs over recent years I am sure that their attitude towards massage therapists is generally a very positive one. Most GPs adopt a policy of wait and see; let the therapist build up his practice and see what the quality of his massage treatments are like and listen to reports from patients and other health professionals.

GPs are obliged under their terms of service to refer patients for services available under the NHS, and referral to massage therapists or any other complementary therapist was not considered as part of the terms of service. Some GPs preferred to suggest that patients visit a particular therapist without actually making a formal referral and may offer to recommend a suitable therapist. However, in doing so they must satisfy themselves that the individual therapist is competent.

The BMA has stated (*Medical Ethics Today*, 1993):

"As a general rule, it is ill-advised for a doctor to refer a patient to any practitioner who is not subject to a registering and disciplinary body."

I am indebted to Joseph Lloyd, L.C.S.P. (Phys.), of Bolton who has passed on to me a copy of a letter from the Policy Officer at the Complementary Therapies Unit of the Department of Health, dated 29th November 2000, which states:

"Remedial massage therapy can be offered on the NHS if local health service commissioners (Primary Care Groups, Health Authorities and Trusts) consider it to be a cost and clinically effective use of resources. Commissioners will also consider if its provision will contribute to the achievement of targets set in the local Health Improvement Programme (HImP). HImP's are set by Health Authorities, who are required to do so in consultation with all those that have an interest in the provision of local health services."

Thus, remedial massage therapists can have a say in their own local arrangements by finding out about the consultation meetings (which are usually published in the local newspapers) and then by attending the meetings and presenting a case for remedial massage in a positive way.

The GP must feel satisfied that the treatment offered by the remedial therapist is appropriate to the patient's needs and is likely to benefit the patient. The GP still retains responsibility for the patient's care and may request that the patient visit the GP's surgery after the remedial massage treatments to review the effects and benefits.

GPs should not be canvassed. It is far better for the therapist to allow his or her treatments to speak for themselves and to build a reputation for the excellence of their treatments and the high professional standards that they apply to their practice.

I had worked in collaboration with many GPs and several consultants during my time as a practitioner. I have found doctors to be fair-minded and supportive and, in many cases, quite enthusiastic about the value of massage treatments, especially for the treatment of low back pain.

I had a contract to work on a regular weekly basis for a group of GPs at their surgery for a period of eighteen months under a government initiative for fund-holding practices to use the treatments of complementary therapists. This scheme was monitored by a team of researchers under the leadership of Judith Emmanuel from the Department of Public Health at Salford University.

The senior partner in the practice told me that, over the years, he had noted the remarks and reactions of his patients who had received treatment at my clinic. When the opportunity arrived under the terms of the scheme that had been introduced into the Health Authority, I was invited to treat patients at the surgery, mainly for acute low back pain and also, on occasions, patients suffering with other musculoskeletal conditions.

The doctors and practice staff were consistently cooperative and I was given full access to all facilities including patient records and reports. My function was to treat patients recommended to me by one or other of the practice partners and, in turn, advise the doctors if I thought any of the patients required further specialised investigation for their condition.

One positive result of this scheme was that the local Health Authority set up a 'bank' of suitably qualified and experienced complementary therapists for the specific purpose of treating low back pain to whom any GP could refer patients at short notice. One of the findings of the research report being that early intervention and treatment by massage (and other therapies, of course) benefited the patient, made earlier recovery more likely with a return to work sooner in most cases. It made good economic sense for the fund-holder practices.

A GP from another practice asked if she could, with the patient's approval, 'sit-in' whilst I treated one of her patients. The patient had a chronic low back problem that gave occasional periods of pain and muscle spasm and the doctor expressed an interest in my method of treatment. The patient came to the clinic and appeared to be in some pain and his body was noticeably bending over to one side.

I treated him by remedial massage to the back and then, as the muscles relaxed, I treated him by passive movements that mobilised his spinal joints and passively stretched the muscles. At the end of the treatment, the patient reported that most of the pain had gone and we could both see that his posture had greatly improved.

At this point the doctor commented that she was able to reduce the patient's pain levels with acupuncture but was unable to get him to stand normally, i.e. straighten him up, and she wanted to see what I was able to do for the patient.

Interestingly enough, she reported that she had completed an acupuncture course accredited by the BMA and that colleagues in her practice had been, to say the least, very dubious about the course and the effects of acupuncture. She used acupuncture on patients suffering from chronic pain and reported a high degree of success in controlling their pain. This reduced the need for continuous pharmaceutical drugs. Not only was this of great benefit to the patients but it made a big difference to the practice finances. She reported wryly that it was at this point that some of her previously sceptical colleagues became much more interested in acupuncture.

Doctors send patients to good remedial massage therapists just as doctors refer to other competent professionals. The therapist must ensure that a professional approach to the patient is adopted, especially in the area of confidentiality. This works in several directions regarding any discussion about the doctor who sends the patient and about other aspects of the patient's treatment. The massage therapist must refrain from commenting upon medical matters, for example, on the diagnosis of a condition by the doctor or aspects of the overall treatment plan that are not his concern but fall within the remit of the GP. Inappropriate comments may confuse and upset the patient and would certainly annoy the doctor who would view it as a serious breach of professionalism.

Chapter 4
Treatment for Specific Areas of the Body

Knee Joint

In the preface to the third edition of, *'Knee Pain and Disability'*, Cailliet (1992) stated that the numbers of people with degenerative conditions of the knee joint has steadily increased in recent years. This, he indicated, is due to several factors including the physical fitness programmes designed to improve general health and cardiovascular fitness resulting in knee problems, the increase in competitive sport and resulting simultaneously multiplied knee injuries, the toll of vehicular accidents and an expanding aged population.

Macnicol (1998) reinforced the views held by Cailliet, referring to the knee as a complex and crucial joint, as easily injured during everyday activities as in sport, industrial accidents or collisions.

The knee has been described as the most poorly protected or exposed joint in the body and as the most frequently injured joint, being involved in a wider variety and larger number of injuries than any other area of the body. Add to this a further statement by Cailliet that the knee joint is probably the most complicated joint in the human body and we begin to understand that knee injuries and knee conditions form a high proportion of the therapist's work.

The principal functions of the knee joint are movement (often rapid and complex) and weight bearing. The joint is often required to perform both functions

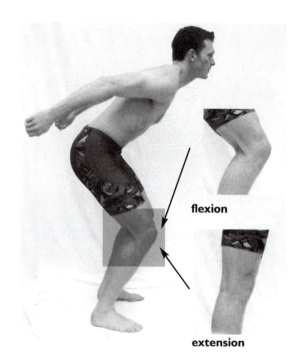

▶ *Figure 22*
The main range
of movement of
the knee joint.

flexion

extension

simultaneously. The joint and its functions are complex and diagnosis, the result of a thorough examination, is the key to successful treatment.

Structure of the Knee Joint

The knee joint is a hinge joint and it is also described as an incongruent joint. The articular bodies of the knee joint consist of the femoral condyles, the tibial condyles and the patella. The incongruency of these surfaces is compensated for by a relatively thick cartilaginous covering, by the menisci, by fatty pads and by the joint fluid. The capsule of the knee joint is wide and lax; thin anteriorly and strengthened by ligaments at the sides.

The fibula corresponds approximately in length to the tibia but is slimmer and more flexible. The proximal fibula articulates with the tibia where it forms an almost immovable synovial joint and is an attachment point for biceps femoris and the lateral collateral ligament. It is known as a compensation joint because, during maximal forward dorsiflexion of the ankle there is expansion of the malleolar joint resulting in compensatory movement in the tibiofibular joint.

The patella is the largest of the sesamoid bones. It is triangular with the tip facing distally. The upper third of the patella serves largely for the attachment of the quadriceps tendon and the lower third serves as the origin for the patellar ligament. The patella has a good covering of protective cartilage, thicker on the posterior surface (facing the femur). Occasionally during palpation the therapist may encounter patella emarginata or patella biparta in which part of the patella appears to be missing or the patella appears to have split into two sections.

The femur is the largest bone in the body. The distal end of the femur forms the knee articulation with tibia and patella. The saddle shaped condyles are separated by a deep, wide fossa and are covered by cartilage to between three and four millimetres. The relationship between tibia and femur is incongruent and assymetrical and does not correspond neatly with each other compared, for example, to the ball and socket of the hip joint. Muscles and ligaments give support and movement and congruity is given by the menisci.

The membranes of the capsule are the synovial and fibrous membranes which are separated by fatty deposits on the anterior and posterior aspects. The capsule is strengthened by the collatoral ligaments. Synovial fluid comes from the fibrous layer of the synovium which is a mesothelium, one of the tissues that line the body. It completely lines the inside of the joint capsule and attaches to each of the bones at the edge of the articular cartilage but it does not cover the weight bearing surfaces of the knee joint.

The fluid produced in the synovium provides lubrication at the joint and contains nutrition for the articular cartilage. The fluid is secreted at the periphery of the joint and is swept into and across the joint by movement.

The menisci of the knee consist of connective tissue and extensive collagen fibre material infiltrated with cartilage-like cells. The collagen fibres run in two principal directions; the strong fibres follow the shape of the menisci between their attachments, that is, to the circumference. The weak fibres pass radially to an imaginary midpoint and interlace between the circumference following fibres. This means that curved, longitudinal tears occur more easily than transverse tears.

The blood supply to an adult meniscus is only to the periphery and they have a very poor repair capability.

The semi-circular medial meniscus is fused with the medial collatoral ligament. The lateral meniscus is almost a closed 'C' shape and it does not fuse with either the capsule or the lateral collateral ligament.

The roles of the menisci include load bearing and impact repulsion, stabilise the knee by keeping the opposing surfaces of femur and tibia apart and help maintain

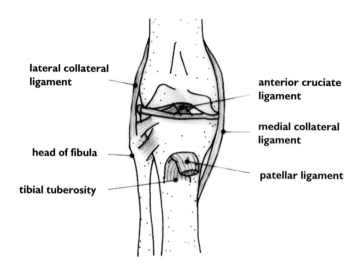

▲ *Figure 23*
Knee joint showing the main ligaments.

correct tensions in capsule and ligaments, and aid lubrication of the joint by exuding synovial fluid and mucin. The menisci are ligamentously attached principally to the tibia, although there are two attachments to the femur by the posterofemoral ligament and the anterior menisciofemoral ligament.

Knee Ligaments

The principal ligaments of the knee include:

1. The patellar ligament which continues from the quadriceps tendon from the lower third of the patella to the tibial tubercle.
2. The medial collatoral ligament which is a flattened trianglar ligament which is built into the capsule of the knee and fused with the medial meniscus. The fibres radiate from the medial epicondyle of the femur to the medial margin of the tibia and into the medial meniscus.
3. The collatoral ligament is not fused with the capsule or the lateral meniscus. It arises from the lateral epicondyle of the femur and attaches to the head of the fibula.
4. The cruciate ligaments occupy the intercondylar notch and are named from their attachments on the tibia, i.e. the anterior tibia and posterior tibia. The cruciates are extra synovial and very strong. Their primary role is to control anterior-posterior movement of the knee.

Knee Examination

It is important to follow the examination procedure; to ask the patient questions and listen carefully to the answers, to examine the patient visually and by palpation and by movements and, if available, any information from other investigations, for example an X-ray report. Ask the patient about his or her symptoms, for example:

- Where does the knee hurt?
- How does it hamper movement?
- Are there any other symptoms?
- Did the patient have knee problems before the present problem?
- Has the patient had any other treatment since injuring the knee?

The therapist should try and establish whether or not the injury is the result of a definite, distinct incident. Generally, if the patient does not remember a specific incident, for example, twisting, giving way to a sharp pain, then it is unlikely that he has suffered a severe injury. If the patient does remember a specific incident the therapist wishes to know more. Was the patient:

- Running straight ahead and in collision with another person or object?
- Turning and perhaps decelerating? This may involve injury to a meniscus or anterior cruciate ligament.
- Involved in an unanticipated movement, for example slipping into a pothole and resulting perhaps in an injury to capsule, ligament or musculotendinous tissue.

I witnessed (along with thirty thousand others) an injury at a premiership football ground some years ago involving a young English international soccer player who passed the ball up field to a colleague and then turned around to take up a new position on the field only for his studs to catch in the turf. The resultant, unanticipated movement did such serious damage to his knee joint that, after much surgery (as reported by Hodkinson, 2000 – eighteen operations) and rehabilitation, the player was forced to retire from the game still in his mid-twenties and with a very noticeable disability of his knee.

Was there sudden eccentric loading of the quadriceps? For example, trying to regain balance when falling can produce enough force to fracture the patella or rupture the patellar ligament. Misjudging a leap can damage the anterior cruciate ligament. Even a mid-air, non-weight bearing incident can produce patella subluxation or injury to the quadriceps group of muscles.

A collision or the introduction of an external force may produce one or all of the 'unholy triad' of injuries to the medial collatoral ligament, medial meniscus and anterior cruciate ligament. This occurs when the force is applied to the lateral aspect of a weight bearing knee and is a common injury in soccer or skiing for example.

The lateral collatoral ligament (and other tissues) may be injured as the result of direct trauma to the medial aspect of the knee. This is a much rarer occurrence than medial knee injuries and such injuries have, in my own particular experience, been in amateur wrestling.

Has the patient experienced direct force on to the anterior aspect of the flexed knee? This used to be referred to as the 'dashboard injury' before car design improved. This type of force may damage the posterior cruciate ligament or may cause fracture and accompanying damage to the patella.

Deceleration and rotation movement of the knee may cause ligament and meniscus damage.

Was the patient aware of any 'noise' from the knee at the time of the incident? If the answer is affirmative, ask the patient to describe the noise. Snapping, tearing, ripping and popping sounds are generally indicative of a severe injury. An injury sound that is audible to someone other than the injured person is certainly an indication of severe injury. A snapping sound or popping sound during deceleration or turning is often an indication of meniscus or anterior cruciate ligament injury.

Other symptoms than pain can help the therapist with his assessment of knee injuries. A patient may complain that the knee either actually gives way unexpectedly or feels as if it is going to give way. Another patient may state that his knee feels as if it is 'bending the wrong way'. Further investigation of the ligaments and meniscus is indicated in both these cases.

'Giving way' was described by Evans (1986) as a neurological phenomenon. This may be caused by local ischaemia to nerves caused by an awkward sitting position that has compressed capillaries supplying the nerves.

The 'giving way' that occurs with meniscal or ligamentous laxity is a reflex phenomenon and is a product of inhibitory impulses caused by pain on the motor neurones at the appropriate spinal level. The muscles switch off and the knee 'gives way'.

In the case of ligament and capsule damage and laxity, the sudden stresses stimulate the Golgi tendon organs and the afferent stimulus acts on the segmental motor neurones, inhibiting nearly all of the muscular activity at the joint. The knee gives way without warning.

Knees often swell when injured. Sometimes the swelling is very rapid and this patient should be referred for prompt expert medical attention, preferably the Accident and Emergency Unit at the local hospital. This rapid swelling may indicate a torn ligament or a fracture.

On other occasions the swelling may be much more gradual or, the patient may inform you, that it has been there for a considerable time.

I can recall several instances over the years when patients presented to me for treatment with knee injuries. On examination these patients were found to be wearing a *Tubigrip* bandage around the injured knee; sometimes doubled over. In each case the bandage had been in place for many weeks or months and had been worn day and night. The knee in question was quite swollen and showed visual evidence of quadriceps muscle atrophy. Now, either the patient had been wrongly advised or had not listened to the correct advice. Whatever the reason, the knee joint was more trouble after such a long confinement in a bandage than the original injury.

A chronic swelling may be due to arthritis and this may have already emerged during the history taking or may become clearer, perhaps, after an X-ray of the knee. Arthritis is the usual reason for what patients describe as 'stiffness' of the knee and they often ascribe this to the effects of old age.

A recently injured knee may be painful and swollen and surrounded by muscles in spasm. The testing must be carried out within the, often limited, pain-free range of movement. Evans (1986) drew attention to the fact that it is helpful to realise that a ruptured ligament is not painful to test because there is nothing to pull on. A severe and multiple ligament injury may be far less painful to examine than a severe sprain.

Do not forget to go over the patient's medical history if this has not been done previously. Not only the history of the patient's knee but also a review of their whole history.

Visual Examination of the Knee

The examination continues with a visual examination and examination by palpation. A full examination stated Apley and Solomon (1997) requires that the therapist be able to see both the patient's legs from groin to toes. The patient should be seen standing and walking, in the sitting position and lying both prone and supine on the examination table. Look at the shape and posture of the lower limbs and see if there is anything unusual; scars, swellings, muscle atrophy, signs of inflammation, fallen arches of the feet. Watch the patient walk to you and away from you. Watch the injured knee during walking to see if it is stable or does it appear to move unnaturally.

Atrophy can be noticed visually by the therapist. However, the patient may be unaware of this and I keep a tape measure handy to measure the circumference of both legs just above the patella. In this way a check that the patient can use and understand will be recorded as the treatments progress and improvement takes place. However, note the statement by Evans on this page.

A normal knee in extension shows clearly the contours of the patella and vastus medialis. There should be well-defined recesses above and on either side of the patella. A swelling, whether blood or synovial fluid, obliterates these spaces, especially on the medial aspect of the knee.

A bursitis at the knee joint, for example a pre-patellar bursa overlying the kneecap, stands out as a sharply demarcated lump, especially when a little gentle pressure is applied to the bursa in question.

Are there any other unusual lumps around the knee joint? These may be cysts or loose bodies, a calcified ligament or, in young patients, a swelling at the tibial tubercle may well be indicative of Osgood-Schlatter's disease.

A visual examination of the posterior knee may show bruising of the calf muscle which, along with knee joint pain, may indicate a posterior cruciate ligament injury.

Swelling around the knee joint should be easily detected in the majority of cases. In the absence of systemic disease or neurological reason, wasting of the quadriceps is, stated Evans (1986), a symptom of trouble in the knee. Wasting may be due to pain inhibition whether this is from the bone in arthritis, the capsule in inflammation or effusion. Wasting may be due to reduced use when the patient 'favours' the good leg. Wasting may also be due to the loss of local reflex arcs, for example, reduced afferent impulses due to tearing or incision of capsular mechanoreceptors or alterations in proprioception due to laxity in the capsular structures. Major injuries or collected minor injuries have a permanent effect on the neurological structures and after some injuries, the quadriceps will not regain their former size despite intensive rehabilitation.

With the patient disrobed to show the whole of each leg, a much more efficient visual examination may be performed rather than a cursory request that the patient rolls up a trouser leg on the affected side.

Palpation of the Knee

After the visual examination, the therapist should feel or palpate the uninjured knee and then the injured knee. Palpation, as we have discussed, is the art of exploring a joint or tissue, mainly by the sense of touch, to discover as much information as possible.

Palpate the uninjured knee and then, using the first palpations as comparisons, explore and discover the secrets of the injured knee. Feel all the major landmarks and start with the obvious – the skin. Check the temperature by feel. Compare the two knees. Progress your hand down from the groin area to the knee; it is normal for the temperature to decrease, to feel slightly cooler as the hand moves to the knee. The therapist should be able to detect changes in warmth.

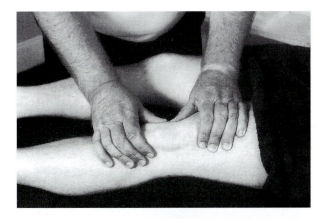

◄ *Figure 24*
Palpation of the patella.

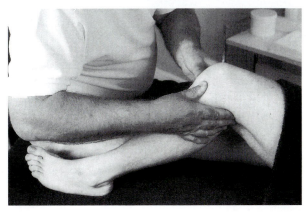

◄ *Figure 25*
Palpation of the
knee in flexion.

Palpation of the synovial membrane was described by Apley and Solomon. A thickened synovial membrane (as in chronic synovitis) can be detected by Solomon's test: grasp the edges of the patella between your thumb and middle finger and try and lift the patella away from the femur. This is not possible but in a healthy knee you have the sense of gripping the patella between your fingers, whereas, if the synovium is thickened, your fingers will simply slip off the edges of the bone.

Palpation always includes feeling for tenderness, locations of pain. Flex both knees within the patient's tolerance and palpate the healthy knee first. Trace around the major landmarks; the actual joint line, the patella, the attachments of the tendons and ligaments. Repeat this on the injured knee and watch the patient's face for any reactions to your touch.

Examination of the Knee by Movements

The therapist already has some indication about the movement of the injured knee; he has watched the patient walk into the examination room and the therapist needs to see how well or how badly the patient can walk and bear weight on the injured knee.

With the patient suitably undressed and towelled on the table I ask him to straighten his leg, i.e. lock out the leg. An inability to do so does not give any conclusive lead but an inability to fully extend the leg may indicate a meniscus or impingement injury to the knee.

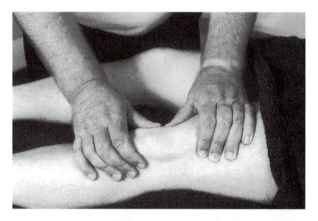

▶ *Figure 26*
Patella movement.

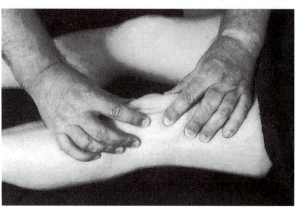

At this point, I add that I pay particular attention to the vastus medialis muscle when examining patients. My experience has shown over the years that a healthy vastus medialis, demonstrated by the patient's ability to sustain a contraction of the muscle for five seconds, is a good indicator of a healthy knee. The inability to sustain a contraction of this muscle is a good indicator of a problem knee. I ask the patient to contract the muscle and I gently but firmly grasp the muscle during the contraction to gauge the strength, or otherwise, of the contraction.

The patella should also be examined at this stage and its movements, superior-inferior and lateral-medial assessed by the therapist. The knee may now be

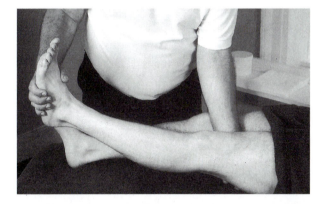

◄ *Figure 27*
(a) Passive extension and;
(b) passive flexion
of the knee.

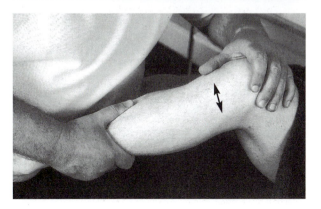

◄ *Figure 28*
Rotation of the tibia.

examined by passive movements into flexion and extension to test for joint integrity. The site(s) of pain and restriction of movement should be noted and returned to later in the examination.

Active movement testing follows; the action of active flexion at the knee tests the hamstring group of muscles and the reverse movement of extension at the knee, tests the quadriceps. If the therapist is not satisfied with the results of the active movements, he may ask the patient to repeat the movements and apply resistance to them. This will make the muscles work very hard until all the muscle fibres

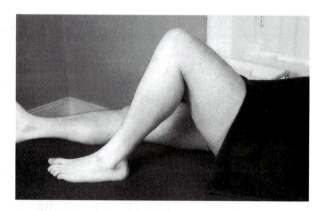

► *Figure 29*
Active flexion of the knee.

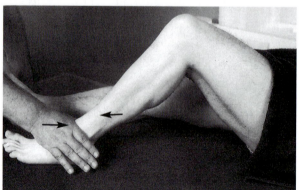

► *Figure 30*
(a) Resisted extension
and;
(b) resisted flexion
of the knee.

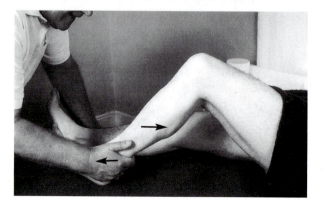

engage in contraction and a thorough 'search' is made of the muscle under the resisted contraction.

There are many more specialised tests for the various structures and tissues that are the province of the medical examiner and the manipulative therapist rather than the remedial massage therapist. The remedial therapist should have enough examination procedures to assess the patient's knee injury and decide which of the tissues is injured. The therapist should also be able to recognise a severe injury, for example a ruptured ligament and to know to make arrangements to get this patient to hospital or to the patient's GP.

Knee Conditions

There are a number of knee conditions that respond well to remedial massage treatment. The therapist must always be aware of any contra-indications to treatment with each patient.

Meniscus Injury

A common injury that occurs more frequently to the medial meniscus than the lateral meniscus. Meniscus injury may occur, for instance, when the knee is in flexion with the foot on the ground and there is an internal rotation of the femur on an abducted and laterally rotated tibia followed by a sudden extension of the knee. The meniscus may be torn by this type of action.

The signs of a meniscus injury include effusion, knee flexed and unable to walk except with weight on forefoot and pain, there may be locking of the knee or giving way at the knee and tenderness at anterior medial aspect of knee. There may be a click as the femoral condyles are moved across a raised meniscal fragment and, in some cases, the click may be painful. Evans pointed out that all clicks do not necessarily come from a meniscus injury and that the meniscus may be normal but may click as it moves over a degenerated articular cartilage. Atrophy of the quadriceps muscles tends to occur quite soon after the damage.

On test the patient is unable to attain full extension of the leg and flexion of the knee is usually limited. There may be crepitus.

Patient on back on table: therapist grasps foot and knee and moves the knee into as full a flexion as possible so that the heel approaches the gluteals. To examine the medial meniscus, the foot is turned outwards whilst the fingers of the other hand compress the postero-medial joint line. From this position the knee is gently extended and the fingers feel for pain and a click at the joint line and the eyes watch the patient's face. This is the McMurray test. To examine the lateral meniscus the foot is held in internal rotation.

Evans warned that diagnosis of a damaged meniscus is never clinically certain and may require arthroscopy to ascertain the exact nature of the problem. Several years ago, I examined a veteran ultra-distance athlete who complained of all the symptoms of a damaged meniscus. Several colleagues concurred as did our GP. She was referred to an orthopaedic consultant who examined the knee and agreed that it was a meniscus problem. A week later, after arthroscopy, the verdict was that the meniscus was intact and there was no evidence of other injury within the knee joint. Eventually a senior massage therapist undertook examination of the knee and found serious problems with the medial hamstring muscles and their attachment to the medial aspect of the knee.

If I suspect a patient has meniscus damage I urge the patient to make an early appointment with his GP with view to further examination and referral. This is because of the poor healing qualities of the meniscus and the intervention of the orthopaedic surgeon will minimise future damage to the joint. Treatment will commence after the investigation by the consultant. The programme will include massage, mobilisation of the joint and stretching and strengthening of the muscles.

Feet, Legs and Ankles

Many conditions that affect the legs are covered in the section of the book that deals with the knee and the hip joints. In the treatment of sports-related injuries the overwhelming proportion of injuries are to the various tissues of the feet, knees, legs and hips.

Foot

The feet are subjected to stress and wear on a daily basis; they are often confined to cramped footwear and punished by the demands of weight bearing and traumatic contact with their environment. Patients complain of pain, difficulty in walking and awkwardness of gait. The muscles that provide movement may be classified into two groups, the:

(a) Extrinsic muscles and;
(b) Intrinsic muscles.

Extrinsic Muscles

The extrinsic muscles of the foot are those that are situated on the lower leg and attach by tendons to the bones of the feet.

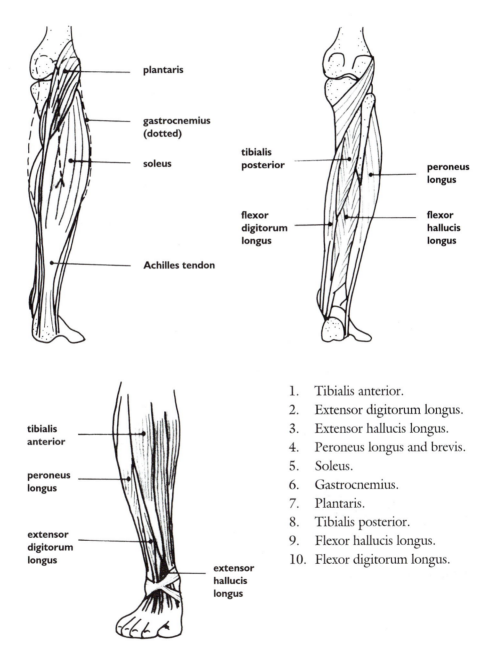

1. Tibialis anterior.
2. Extensor digitorum longus.
3. Extensor hallucis longus.
4. Peroneus longus and brevis.
5. Soleus.
6. Gastrocnemius.
7. Plantaris.
8. Tibialis posterior.
9. Flexor hallucis longus.
10. Flexor digitorum longus.

▲ *Figure 31*
The lower leg illustrating the extrinsic muscles of the foot.

These muscles have a variety of functions that include:

1. Plantar and dorsiflexion of the foot.
2. Inversion and eversion.
3. Maintenance of the arch of the foot.

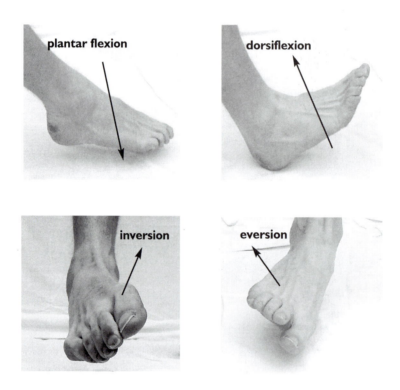

▲ *Figure 32*
Various functions of the foot include;
(a) plantar flexion; (b) dorsiflexion; (c) inversion; (d) eversion.

Intrinsic Muscles of the Foot

The origins and the insertions of the intrinsic muscles are found within the foot itself. Their major function is that of 'cupping' the sole of the foot and a source of strength to the natural longitudinal arch. The muscles work on the toes and provide their movements. Some of these are described by their Latin names, for example:

1. Flexor digitorum brevis.
2. Abductor hallucis.

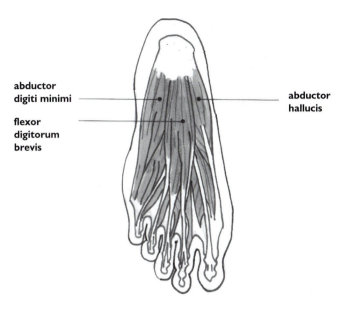

▲ *Figure 33*
Intrinsic muscles of the foot.

The muscles are all covered by the plantar aponeurosis that is derived from the plantar fascia which originates from the calcaneal tuberosity. It splits anteriorly at the metatarsophalangeal joints to allow flexor tendons access to their insertions. A section of plantar fascia proceeds to the base of the fifth metatarsal head and forms part of the spring ligament.

There are no muscles on the dorsum of the foot. The tendons of some of the extrinsic muscles pass along the dorsum of the foot as they travel to their insertions.

Examination of the Foot and Ankle

The examination procedure for patients with foot and ankle injuries follows the same outline as for other conditions.

Firstly, the patient is encouraged to describe their injury and how and when it happened. Find out about the pain, any difficulties and awkwardness of gait that the patient reports. For instance, a history of cramps when walking that are relieved by rest may suggest a problem with arterial blood supply. This patient should be referred either to the GP or to a qualified and experienced podiatrist for further examination. The therapist goes through the patient's medical history.

The patient should then expose his legs at least from the knee down for the remainder of the examination. Foot pain may occur while standing or walking and the patient should be examined whilst standing and walking, too. There are criteria for a normal foot that should be kept in mind during the examinations:

1.   The foot should normally be free of pain;
2.   There should be good muscle balance;
3.   There should be an absence of contracture, e.g. an abnormally high arch;
4.   In both standing and walking the heel should be central, not deviating to one side or the other;
5.   The toes should be straight and mobile;
6.   Whilst standing and in the stance phase of walking there should be three sites of weight bearing – the first and the fifth metatarsal heads and the calcaneum.

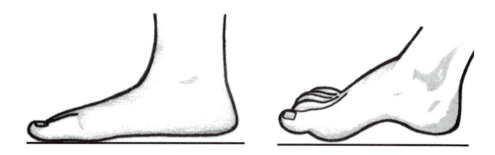

▲ *Figure 34*
Two common types of foot shape;
(a) pes planus and; (b) pes cavus.

There are also a variety of foot shapes:

1.   Pes rectus. A normal healthy foot with balanced load bearing and a lower lateral malleolus.
2.   Pes planus. A flat foot in which the plantar arch has disappeared due to inadequacies of the intrinsic muscles and over-extension of the ligaments. This causes pronation of the talus that slides medially and other tarsal bones shift positions. Pain can occur in lower leg due to pressures on extrinsic muscles and tendons.
3.   Pes varus. Also known as 'club foot' and caused by paralysis or damage to peroneals, extensor digitorum longus or extensor hallucis longus resulting in oversupination.
4.   Pes valgus. A pronated or everted foot.
5.   Pes planovalgus. A combination of flat foot and overpronation with the foot bulging medially and calcaneum pronated.
6.   Pes cavus. A high arched foot.

Examination in the Standing Position

In a standing position, the therapist:

1. Looks for any disclouration, swelling or deformity.
2. Checks for weak or fallen arches.
3. Asks the patient to walk normally.
4. Asks the patient to stand on tiptoes and, if possible, walk on tiptoes.
5. Checks that the gait is smooth and the foot well balanced?

Does the patient walk on the outer edge of the foot or does he walk on the medial edge? Have a look at the patients' shoes for any wear patterns that may be linked to how they walk.

There is great value in taking the footprint of the patient's standing foot on a sheet of paper. It helps the patient understand the therapist's explanation.

In the case of runners with foot injuries I always request that they bring at least one pair of well-used running shoes with them. The wear patterns can give excellent pointers to the patient's problem and have good diagnostic value about the presenting condition, for example:

1. The normal foot should show slight wear on the outside of the heel;
2. A drop foot due to muscle weakness scuffs the toe;
3. Worn areas towards the front of the sole may indicate relative problems with metatarsal heads.

Examination in the Lying Position

Now ask the patient to lie on the examination table and take a closer look at both feet. Examine the toes, look at the skin especially for any thickening in the form of corns or calluses. Any redness or bruising visible?

Palpate the feet and feel for any changes in temperature. Feel for any swellings, tenderness or any abnormal sensation that the patient may report. Feel the dorsum of the foot for any painful areas and check the tendons and insertions.

Move the ankle into dorsi- and plantar flexion. Do this with the leg straight and then with the leg flexed and see if there is any difference in the patient's reactions. Grasp the calcaneum and move the foot into inversion and eversion. Check the movements of the joints of the toes.

Ankle problems and injuries occur commonly, with perhaps the lateral ankle sprain being most common. Look for swelling and disclouration around the injured joint and feel the bony landmarks, the tendons and, of course, the ligaments. The therapist will already have picked up much information about the patient's ankle injury and examination by movement will be restricted to active and gentle passive movements to ascertain the exact site of injury.

Treatment of Foot and Ankle Conditions

The remedial massage therapist can treat many foot and ankle conditions successfully by massage and mobilising techniques. However, there will be many occasions when the patient requires more expert examination and treatment.

Many years ago I made a valuable contact with Phil Laxton, a senior tutor at the then Northern College of Chiropody based at Salford College of Technology, now with University status bestowed. The college accepted referrals from remedial massage therapists as well as other health professionals. The more complicated the problems the more interested they were.

The patients were given appointments for a full biomechanical examination by a small group of students under the supervision of a tutor. The findings of the examination were always sent to me in the mail. In most cases, remedial action was taken by the students under the direction and supervision of the tutor and treatments began immediately. Many patients enjoyed expensive and successful treatments at little or no cost to them.

I referred patients with congenital conditions that caused, in some cases, distressing physical, psychological and social problems. Sportsmen and women of international rank as well as weekend participants went along. Members of the public with a selection of foot and ankle injuries that required more specialised examination and treatment than I could offer were, 'sent to Salford'.

I greatly valued the association with the college. On occasions I accompanied my patients and was welcomed as a fellow practitioner and discussed my patients with the tutors and students. I also learned a lot about feet and gait, about orthotics, supports, taping and strapping. My patients thanked me for obtaining expert help for them and, more often than not, I continued to treat the patients anyway.

With my experiences in mind, I urge my students to make contact with the nearest chiropody and podiatry college and benefit from the help offered by their clinics and the expertise of the tutors.

Foot and Ankle Massage

Contrast Bathing

Contrast bathing is the use of hot and cold water to bathe a part of the body for therapeutic effect. It is better used after the acute stage of an injury has passed and feet and ankles lend themselves better than most parts of the body to this treatment. It is an excellent self-help treatment for anyone with tired feet from too much standing about or too much walking.

Ideally the patient will have two bowls of water. One filled with hot water of about the same temperature as when washing ones face and certainly no hotter. The second bowl is filled with ordinary water from the cold water tap. There is no need to add ice to the cold water.

The patient places the foot into the hot water for three minutes. After this time has elapsed, the foot is taken out of the warm water and placed in the cold water for one minute. This procedure is repeated until the patient has experienced both the hot and cold three times. The session is now completed with a final session in the hot water bowl.

To complement this treatment the patient should rest on a settee or bed for an hour or so with the injured side elevated. The stimulation to the circulation from the contrast bathing will be aided by the gravitational drainage of the elevation.

Metatarsalgia

Metatarsalgia, or pain in the matatarsals, is a common condition. The main symptom is pain in the area of the metatarsal heads often described as severe and burning by many sufferers. Some patients claim they have to sleep with the foot outside the bedclothes in an effort to cool the burning.

Usually, the problem is that the second, third and fourth metatarsal heads have dropped and have begun to take the weight that is normally supported by the first and fifth metatarsal heads; the weight-bearing triangle.

Causes

This may be due to weakening in the supportive muscles due to illness; straining of the supportive muscles, possibly due to an increase in body weight; or straining these muscles due to a change in working habits, for example, long periods of standing or carrying heavy weights. In women the wearing of high-heeled shoes is thought to contribute to this problem.

Examination

On checking the plantar surface of the foot, the therapist will probably find that the inner three metatarsal heads will bulge slightly instead of there being an arch. Pressure applied to the fourth metatarsal head will produce pain. The smaller toes will tend to become plantar flexed and may develop corns over the proximal phalangeal joints. In long-term cases periostitis will have developed in the shafts of the metatarsals near the anterior heads and there could be traumatic arthritis of the metatasophalangeal joints.

Treatment

The first aim of treatment is the relief of pain. Place a pad of chiropody felt under the three inner metatarsal heads that will automatically raise them. Using taping to secure the pad in place and by applying the taping in a downward direction from the dorsum of the foot, pull down the first and fifth metatarsal heads to their normal position. This will encourage the arch into its correct position as well as relieve the painful symptoms.

The pad and taping should be kept in place for about ten days. If the examination shows that there are corns present the patient should be referred to a chiropodist for appropriate treatment.

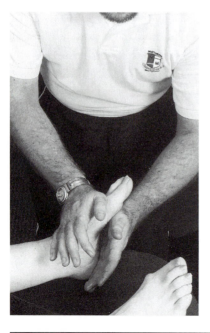

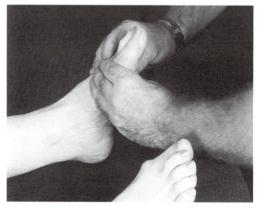

◄▲ *Figure 35*
Hand positions for foot massage on metatarsals.

After ten days the patient is treated by a thorough foot massage to reduce swelling, break down any adhesions, restore some flexibility and stimulate the circulation. Deep frictions and bone shaking should be included in the treatment.

Use of a faradic foot bath for between ten and fifteen minutes with a strong current is beneficial at this treatment.

The foot should now be re-padded for a further ten days after which there should be three intensive massage treatments in seven days. During this time the pad and taping are left off but after the third of these treatments the pad and taping are re-applied for a further ten days until another massage treatment. In most cases the problems have eased after this final treatment and the patient can disregard the padding and taping.

Stress Fractures of the Foot

Stress fractures may occur in anyone and are usually the result of prolonged and repeated loading, for example in long distance runners, intensive trainers in other sports and those who are poorly conditioned or poorly prepared for the activities or event in which they participate. The most common sites are the calcaneum, the navicular and the metatarsals.

The symptoms are localised pain on activity, tenderness on palpation and localised swelling. An X-ray will confirm the presence of a stress fracture once the healing process takes place in the bone and a scan will be more productive.

The treatment is mainly by keeping the weight bearing off the injured foot and by rest, thus allowing the bone to heal quickly and normally. Some massage above the site of the injury may be given and, once healing has completed, a thorough massage of the foot can be undertaken.

It would be opportune to discuss the problem with the patient and get them to re-assess their activities or training schedules and also to investigate the suitability of footwear and equipment, thus preventing future problems.

Hallux Valgus and Hallux Rigidus

These are two conditions that painfully affect the big toe and in agreeing to undertake treatment of patients with these conditions I would collaborate with the patient's podiatrist.

Hallux Valgus

This is a deviation of the big toe towards the smaller ones. It tends to be progressive and fluid in the bursa over the first metatarsophalangeal joint becomes inflamed and results in a bunion. Additional discomfort may be brought about to the patient by the appearance of a corn that forms the centre of the bunion and can give severe pain. The cause of this condition is the failure of the muscles that keep the big toe in alignment:

1.   Flexor hallucis brevis and longus.
2.   Extensor hallucis brevis and longus.
3.   Adductor hallucis.

Provided the muscles are balanced and there are no other factors involved the big toe will remain in line.

If something causes the adductor hallucis tendon to weaken and lengthen and other muscles tighten and shorten, the big toe will be forced towards the smaller toes and hallux valgus begins.

As the big toe deviates, the metatarsal splays outward to form the medial projection which is characteristic of this condition. Pressure of footwear against this projection will produce, in turn, tenderness, inflammation, callous formation, adventitious bursa, corn and bunion.

The condition may be triggered by shoes with narrow and pointed toes, tight and pointed stockings or tights, a splay-foot walk, i.e. with the feet at the 'ten minutes to two' position or even heredity may be a factor.

Severe and chronic cases may only be successfully helped by surgery due to the onset of arthritis in the joint and the amount of inflammation and fibrous tissue build-up around the joint.

In the early stages the condition can be helped by twice weekly massage of the foot with mobilisation of the joint. Electrotherapy in the form of ultrasound or interferential is a further option for treatment. The toes may also be trained back into alignment by the application of a taping to exert a continuous and steady pressure to pull the big toe away from the smaller ones.

Hallux Rigidus

The big toe becomes rigid because the first metatarsophalangeal joint will not dorsi- or plantar flex. The condition is usually of traumatic onset and affects one side only.

The patient may have stubbed the toe on a raised flagstone or had something heavy dropped on the toe causing bruising and bleeding into the joint. In non-traumatic cases, the condition is usually associated with conditions like pes planus that imposes a severe long-term strain upon the joint. The joint becomes chronically inflamed, the capsule becomes rigid and movement ceases, with the exception of a little plantar flexion in most cases.

Because there is no dorsiflexion, the push-off phase in walking may mean walking over on to the tip of the toe (causing even more strain) or the foot may be rotated and the inner side of the toe is used to push-off.

The worse cases of hallux rigidus will require surgery. However, if the condition is treated early enough, many patients can be helped considerably by massage of the whole foot, frictions around the joint, simple traction movements and then passive plantar and dorsiflexion movements.

Children with Foot Conditions

We do not expect children to suffer from the foot conditions experienced by adults apart from the occasional minor traumatic injury. Any child who experiences foot pain or problems with walking should be referred to the GP who in turn will probably pass the child on to the appropriate expert.

Some children develop a condition known as Apophysitis Calcanei in which the Achilles tendon attachment to the calcaneum becomes fragmented. This is often the result of overloading and the strong musculotendinous stress on a weaker bony attachment.

The child experiences pain on walking and running and soreness and stiffness at rest. A limp develops and swelling over the calcaneum. It is tender on palpation. The child must be referred to his or her GP.

The GP may be willing for the therapist to treat the child under his supervision and treatment consists of rest from all strenuous or painful activity. The use of a temporary heel pad to relieve pressure; massage of the foot and calf muscles; cooling the injured area with cold packs or the use of an anti-inflammatory gel like *Enzyme Ice* will be beneficial and effective.

Lateral Ankle Sprain

This injury is suffered by most people at least once in their lifetime. For a period of time in the late 80's and early 90's I was the masseur to the English Fell Running team and lateral ankle sprains – and their long-term effects – were very common amongst the runners.

The ankle does not have to be grossly swollen in the acute stage to be seriously injured. Care should be taken during the examination process for this injury. I remember beginning to examine a dancer with such an injury and without a second thought I passively took her injured foot in to eversion and inversion to test movement and the poor patient fainted with the pain.

Examination, therefore, should be thorough and careful and in some cases the therapist may decide to refer the patient directly to the Accident and Emergency Department of the local hospital for a more detailed examination and X-ray to determine the degree of damage and check for fracture.

The patient will be in pain, and usually have a visible swelling and restriction of movement at the injured joint. There may be periosteal damage including an avulsion fracture at the attachment of the ligament. The anterior talofibular ligament is commonly injured in this type of ankle trauma and produces a swelling, noticeably in front of the lateral malleolus. The calcaneofibular ligament produces pain and swelling distal to the lateral malleolus.

The deltoid ligament features in a much smaller percentage of injuries and occurs in overpronation injuries or when the foot is turned out violently. This injury gives tenderness and swelling below the medial malleolus. Treatment in the **acute stage** consists of:

- Massage above the site of injury to encourage drainage away from the site;
- Ice every two hours during the next twenty-four hours for fifteen minutes. This can be re-assessed later;
- The patient is required to rest from aggravating activities;
- Elevation of the ankle will be helpful, especially during the resting period;
- I would recommend the use of *Enzyme Ice* and both *Ruta Grav* and *Arnica* in tablet form at this stage but later in cream form;
- Stabilisation of the joint by strapping and padding.

Treatment in the **sub-acute** stage consists of:

- Massage of the foot and lower leg;
- Gentle passive movements of the injured joint;
- Ultrasound (which may be used initially in treatment);
- Continue with the strapping support for about seven days and then re-assess;
- Gentle active exercises, i.e. ankle movements within pain threshold;
- Contrast bathing.

Treatment in the **chronic stage** consists of:

- Continue with massage to foot and lower leg;
- Frictions across the ligament(s);
- Ultrasound;
- Contrast bathing;
- Active movements and partial weight bearing.

Recovery Period

In a healthy young adult with no other complicating factors the healing period for this injury is about twelve weeks. Pushing the patient too quickly or a lack of understanding of the injury will lead to chronic problems with laxity of the joint. It would be a good idea to use supportive strapping when the patient returns to activity or training. The strapping may also be used as a preventative measure in future competition and hard training – provided it is applied in the correct way by someone who knows what they are doing and why they are doing it.

Shoulder

The shoulder is a beautiful joint and it is also rather complicated. For instance, depending upon which text you read, the shoulder consists of five joints or even seven joints (Cailliet, 1971).

Common usage refers to the glenohumeral joint as the shoulder joint. However it is only one of a number of joints that form the shoulder complex. All of the joints are separately and collectively important in normal shoulder function and injury or impairment of one of the joints may cause impairment of all the joints in the complex.

The joints of the shoulder complex move synchronously, each depending upon the others and dysfunction resulting from injury to any one of the joints affects the function of the remaining joints. Shoulder movement takes place by synchronised movements occurring simultaneously in a smooth, integrated manner which was described by Codman (1934) as the scapulohumeral rhythm. Thus examination of the shoulder should include an examination of each joint as well as the collective movement.

Joints of the Shoulder Complex

1. The glenohumeral joint.
2. The suprahumeral joint.
3. The acromioclavicular joint.
4. The scapulocostal joint.
5. The costosternal joint.
6. The sternoclavicular joint.
7. The costovertebral joint.

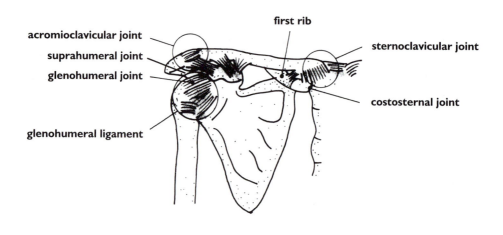

▲ *Figure 36*
Some joints of the shoulder complex.

The suprahumeral joint is not perhaps a joint in the true sense of the word, i.e. not an articulation between two bones. It is more a protective articulation between the head of the humerus and an arch formed by a broad triangular ligament connecting the acromial and caracoid processes. The suprahumeral joint prevents trauma from above to the glenohumeral joint or head of the humerus and also prevents upward dislocation of the humerus. The glenoid cavity, acromion process, caracoid process and the coracoidal ligament are the 'sides' of the joint with the humeral head lying under this protective covering. Many important and sensitive tissues are found within this small area:

1. Part of the subacromial bursa.
2. Subcoracoid bursa.
3. Supraspinatus muscle and tendon.
4. Superior portion of the joint capsule.
5. Portion of the biceps tendon.

As the arm abducts, the greater tuberosity of the humerus must pass under the coracromial ligament and not compress the enclosed tissues. This movement requires fine muscular coordination. Impairment will result in pain and limitation of movement.

The glenohumeral joint (commonly referred to as the shoulder joint) is a classic incongruous joint. The surfaces of the joint are not symmetrical or parallel with the opposing concave and convex surfaces equidistant.

The convex surface is roundly cylindrical. The larger convex portion does not seat itself in the smaller shallow concave portion. The movement is not rotational about a fixed axis but more of a gliding movement about a constantly changing axis. Movement and stability at this joint are supplied by musculature.

Shoulder Movement

The shoulder is more prone to dislocation than most joints. It is a very mobile joint and lacks stability. To perform the movement of circumduction requires the combined effort of some twenty-nine muscles.

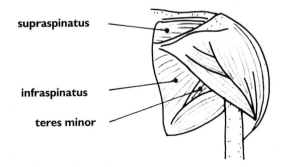

supraspinatus

infraspinatus

teres minor

◀ *Figure 37*
The rotator cuff
(S.I.T.S) muscles
(the subscapularis
is anterior and has
not been illustrated).

Perhaps the best known of the shoulder muscles that act upon the glenohumeral joint are the musculotendinous cuff muscles, also known as the rotator cuff muscles or simply by their initials, the S.I.T.S. muscles. They are:

1.   Supraspinatus.
2.   Infraspinatus.
3.   Teres minor.
4.   Subscapularis.

Shoulder Examination

Shoulder examination follows the same procedures as other examinations and the therapist should begin by obtaining the patient's subjective account of his or her injury and then the patient's medical history. The therapist should also be aware that pain may be referred to the shoulder area by other conditions, for example, from the cervical spine or the heart.

The visual examination also begins as soon as the therapist meets the patient and, more formally, the patient should expose both shoulders, neck, upper limbs and be examined from the front, the sides and the back. The therapist looks for any visible signs that may help in the assessment of the patient. This will include:

*   Any scars, lumps, bruising or discolouration;
*   Symmetry of the shoulders;
*   'Winging' of the scapulae;
*   Wasting of the deltoid;
*   Acromioclavicular dislocation;
*   Joint swelling;
*   Wasting or tightness of the pectoral muscles;
*   Effusion into the axilla.

How do the arms hang? For example there may be an internal rotation of one arm that may indicate a posterior dislocation.

The therapist progresses to an examination by palpation, to feel the joints of the shoulder, e.g. the clavicles, acromion processes, acromioclavicular joints, head of the humerus on either side, around the scapulae. Explore the muscles and their attachments where possible.

Examination by movements is carried out by; active, passive and resisted movements as outlined below. The therapist examines for limitation of movement and for pain and should bring the examination to a conclusion whenever a positive reaction is experienced by the patient.

Examination of the Shoulder by Active Movements

The therapist may stand in front of the patient and demonstrate the movements he requires the patient to perform. However, the therapist may also need to look at some of the movements from other vantage points.

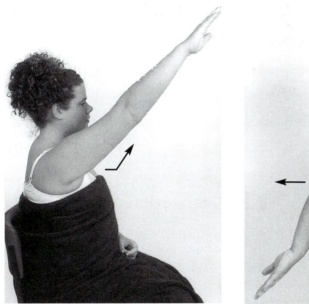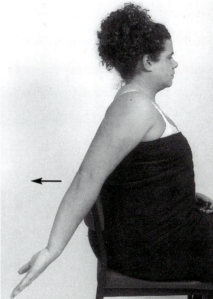

▲ *Figure 38*
(a) Active flexion and; (b) active extension of the shoulder.

Active flexion and active extension of the arm, i.e. the patient takes the arm out in front and upwards and then takes the arm down and backwards.

Active abduction, i.e. away from the body and upward followed by active adduction when the patient returns the arm to the body.

Perhaps the best way to examine the movements of internal and external rotation is for the patient to flex the elbow to ninety degrees with the upper arm parallel to the body. The patient is then instructed to move the arm away from the body into lateral rotation and then to move the arm back and across the chest into medial rotation.

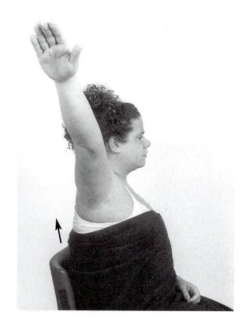

▶ *Figure 39*
Active abduction
of the shoulder.

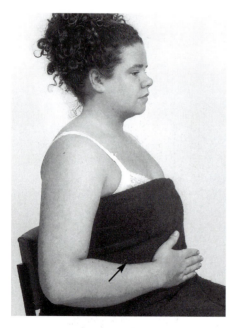

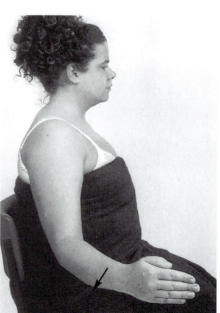

▲ *Figure 40*
(a) Active medial rotation and; (b) active lateral rotation of the shoulder.

Having progressed through these movements without discomfort the patient may be requested to perform the movement of circumduction anteriorly and then posteriorly, that is by making big circles with their arms in both directions to give a picture of the total shoulder movement.

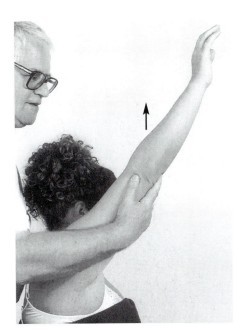
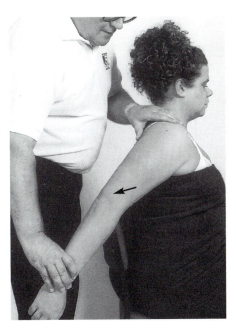

▲ Figure 41
(a) Passive flexion and; (b) passive extension of the shoulder.

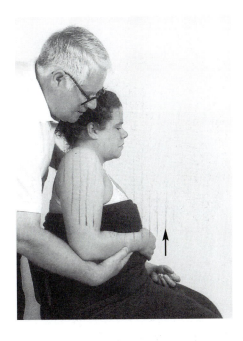
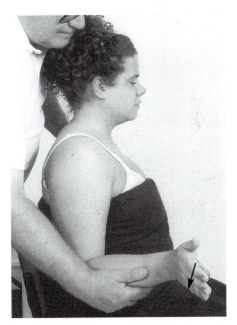

▲ Figure 42
(a) Passive medial rotation and; (b) passive lateral rotation of the shoulder.

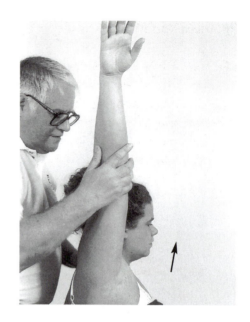

▶ *Figure 43*
Passive abduction and
elevation of the shoulder.

Examination of the Shoulder by Passive Movements

If there have been no painful or other significant reactions to the examination by active movements, the same movements may be carried out by the therapist holding the patient's arm. I do not include circumduction in the passive examination of the shoulder.

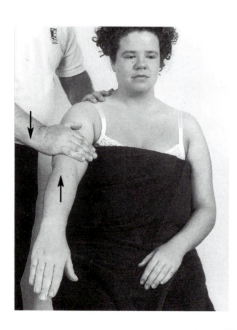

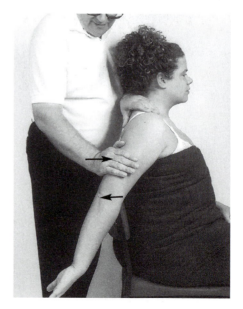

▲ *Figure 44*
(a) Resisted flexion and; (b) resisted extension of the shoulder.

Examination of the Shoulder by Resisted Movements

The therapist may, on occasions, need to examine the patient's shoulder movements by adding resistance to the active movements described above. The patient is requested to move the shoulder actively in to the movements of flexion, extension, abduction, adduction, lateral and medial rotation. To each separate movement the therapist applies resistance, just enough to make the patient use the muscles of the shoulder quite hard but not applying too much resistance that would block movement completely. In this way, all the fibres of the muscles are required to work hard and even small muscle injuries, if they exist, will cause a reaction in the patient.

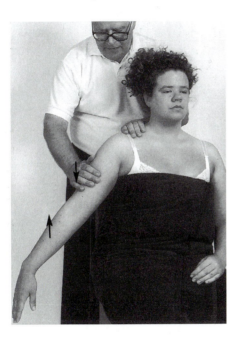

◀ *Figure 45*
Resisted abduction
of the shoulder.

Treatment of the Neck and Shoulders

Massage of the neck and shoulders has much benefit for just about everyone. It is in this area that stress and tension manifest their physiological symptoms. The stress of everyday living affects us all, very often on a daily basis. Hans Selye, in the 30's, talked about "distress" rather than "stress" and he and fellow researchers outlined the major causes of stress that included the following:

- Moving house.
- Travel, especially by air.
- Looming examinations.
- Driving tests.

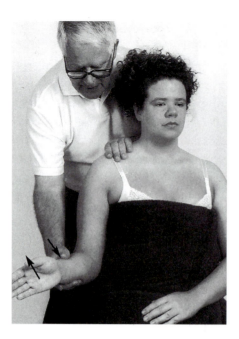 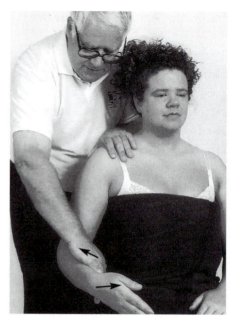

▲ Figure 46
(a) Resisted lateral rotation and; (b) resisted medial rotation of the shoulder.

- Personal long-term illness.
- Long-term illness in the household.
- Death of a loved one.
- Financial problems.
- Working conditions/relationships.
- Breakdown of personal relationship.
- Environmental stresses.
- Noisy neighbours.
- Crime and vandalism.
- Civil unrest and war.

This list is not complete but it will give the reader an idea of the causes of stress and tension which transfers partly to the musculoskeletal structures and to the neck area in particular.

The neck and shoulders are also prone to other types of injuries, for example, the commonly termed 'whiplash' syndrome associated with some road traffic accidents. Torticollis or 'wry neck' associated with exposure to a cold draft. Strains, even sprains, brought on by poor posture, or work induced injuries. Office workers with twenty or thirty years experience may present with quite complicated neck and shoulder symptoms due to poor working posture. Players of

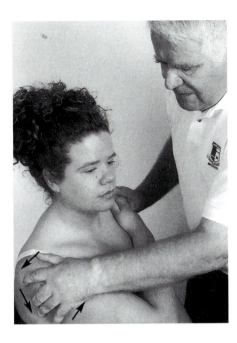

◄ *Figure 47*
Rotation movement of
the patient's left shoulder.

some sports, for example rugby players or amateur wrestlers are liable to suffer neck injury. People who drive for a living are also at risk.

Muscles may become hypertonic and occasionally may develop a painful spasm. The muscle problem then has a knock-on effect to the joints and their tissues. Joints may become misaligned by the constant pressure exerted by the hypertonic muscle. It has been suggested that this may be the cause of osteoarthritis in the cervical joints.

Pain may be referred from the neck into the shoulder, the arm, or the hand due to compression or pressure on a nerve pathway as it emerges from the upper thoracic or lower cervical spine. Not only pain may result but also loss of function in some cases.

Examination of the Neck

The therapist must follow the procedures outlined in the section about examination of the patient, when dealing with every new patient.

Thus, the patient should be seated and asked questions about the current problem with the neck/shoulders and the answers noted by the therapist. This questioning continues with the task of eliciting the patient's full medical history to the current time.

During the examination process the therapist carries out a continuous visual examination of the patient but now moves to a more specific examination of the neck and shoulder area. For this the patient should be allowed to remove their upper garments behind the screen and be given a towel to wrap around the upper body. (Female patients are not required to remove the bra during examination or treatment).

The therapist now undertakes a specific and detailed visual examination of the patient, remembering, of course, that the patient is three-dimensional and needs to be examined from the back, front and both sides. During this visual examination the therapist looks for anything which he considers to be out of the ordinary, to look for balance of posture and symmetry of arms and shoulders. Is the patient's neck on straight or is there an incline to one side or the other? Make a note of any abnormality of the cervical and thoracic curves.

The next step is to examine by palpation of the tissues of the neck and shoulders. Start, in the case of a shoulder problem, with the uninjured side before moving to the injured shoulder. Is there a difference in temperature? Does your exploratory probing cause pain or discomfort to the patient. Feel into the bony landmarks around the scapulae and the acromioclavicular joints, the head of the humerus as it nears the glenoid. Palpate the muscles that are available, for example, deltoids, pectoralis insertion into the humerus, the muscular attachments around the scapulae and from the scapulae to the vertebrae, e.g. the rhomboids, levator scapulae, and the superficial muscle that lies like a scarf just below the skin, trapezius. Search the attachments around the base of the skull, the neck and shoulder around to the clavicle and down the spines of the scapulae to the 12th thoracic vertebra. These palpatory investigations yield fruitful information about the patient.

The patient may now be examined by movement of the shoulder joint and/or the neck. Ask the patient to demonstrate the range of movement they have within their pain threshold. This gives the examiner a good idea about the pain the patient feels and how much movement the patient appears to have.

This is followed by a passive examination of the affected area, i.e. the movements are carried out by the therapist upon the patient.

Examination of the Neck by Passive Movements

The purpose here is to find out if there is an injury to any of the cervical joints. The patient is seated and the therapist stands behind the patient. Before starting this examination, it is wise to remove spectacles, earrings and hearing aids from the patient.

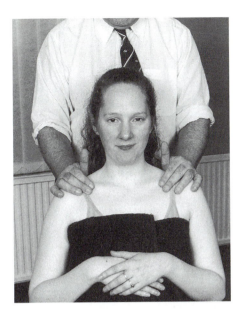

◄ *Figure 48*
Use of the therapist's thumbs in
the neck movement examination.

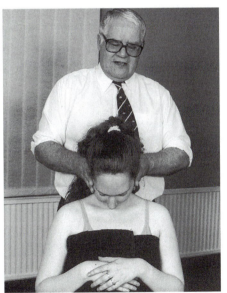

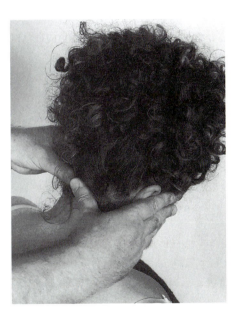

▲ *Figure 49*
Forward flexion of the neck – note the thumbs just below the occipital bone.

To start the examination by passive movements, the therapist holds the patient's head in both hands; it is cradled by the hands along the side of the head and the thumbs just below the occipital bone.

From this position the patient is taken slowly into forward flexion of the neck and asked to comment upon the movement for pain, ease of movement.

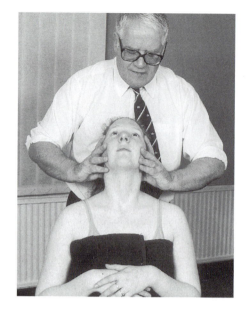

▶ *Figure 50*
The patient's neck being
extended towards the ceiling.

This is followed by a steady movement into extension so that the patient is looking directly up to the ceiling. As the movement progresses the therapist must be alert for the sudden appearance of symptoms like pain, cessation of movement, crepitus. This movement is naturally limited by the bony vertebral joints.

By a slight adjustment of the hands to the sides of the patient's head, the therapist now side turns the patient's head to the right and to the left. Each movement must be done slowly and with care. The range of movement in each direction should be noted and, of course, any painful reaction by the patient.

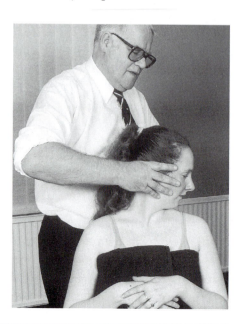

▶ *Figure 51*
Passive side turn of the neck
to the patient's left.

From the same position, the therapist carries out side bending of the patient's neck to the right and then to the left. Again the range and quality of the movement should be noted and any other symptoms experienced by the patient.

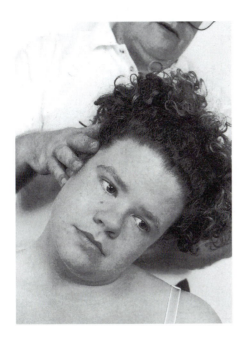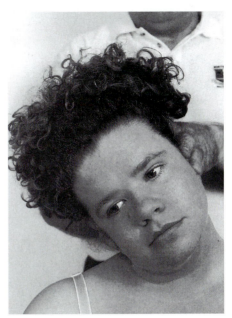

▲ *Figure 52*
(a) Passive side bend to the right and; (b) passive side bend to the left of the neck.

At the conclusion of the examination by passive movements the therapist should be able to note any pain, stiffness or limitation in the movements of the cervical vertebrae. Depending upon what, if anything, the examination by passive movements shows up, the therapist may progress to the examination by active movements.

Examination of the Neck by Active Movements

Active movements are the movements performed by the patient using their own muscles and the objectives of this examination are to ascertain the health and strength of the muscles that move the neck.

The therapist stands in front of the patient to start this sequence and may demonstrate to the patient exactly what movement is required.

Firstly the patient is asked to move the neck into forward flexion. At the end of the range of movement and provided there is no adverse reaction to the

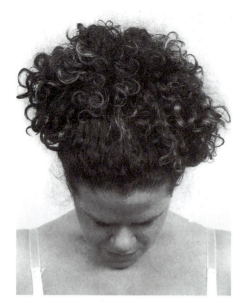
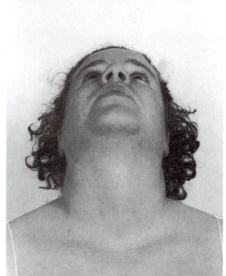

▲ *Figure 53*
(a) Active flexion and; (b) active extension of the neck.

movement of flexion, the patient is now asked to extend the neck by slowly looking up towards the ceiling. The therapist monitors the range of active movements and asks the patient if any pain or discomfort has been experienced whilst performing the movement.

At this stage of the examination, my preference is to move and stand behind the patient. Place both hands flat on either side of the patient's neck with the thumbs

▶ *Figure 54*
The therapist uses the thumbs to estimate the range of active side bend.

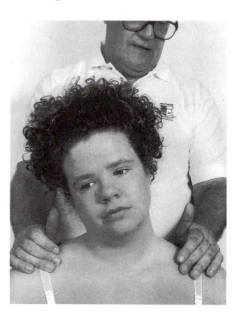

raised and pointing towards the ceiling. The two thumbs are in position to act as indicators of the range of movement. The patient is requested to side bend the neck firstly to the right and then towards the left. The patient is asked if there has been any pain or discomfort experienced. The therapist has an indication of the range of movement by how closely the head moved towards the extended thumbs in each movement.

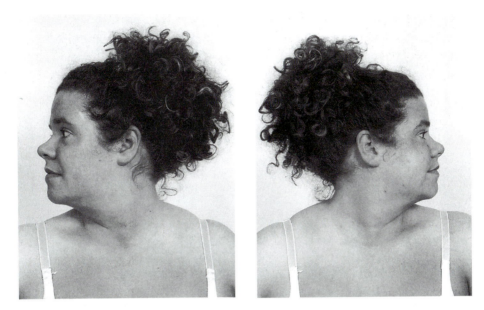

▲ *Figure 55: (a) Active side turn to the right and; (b) active side turn to the left of the neck.*

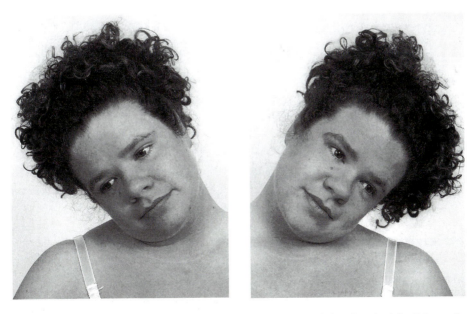

▲ *Figure 56: (a) Active side bend to the right and; (b) active side bend to the left of the neck.*

The same manoeuvre with the thumbs used as a guide to range of movement is repeated with the movements of active side bending to the right and then to the left. The therapist gauges the range and quality of the movement and asks the patient about any pain or discomfort caused by the movements.

Examination of the Neck by Resisted Movements

These movements are usually enough to search out any muscle or joint problems with the neck. Occasionally, the therapist may need to take the examination a step further and examine the range of movements by applying some resistance as the patient moves through the active range of movements. For example, the movements of flexion, extension, side bending and side turning are performed by the patient against the resistance of the therapist's hands.

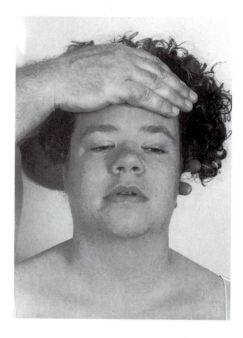

▶ *Figure 57*
Resisted extension of the neck.

At the conclusion of the stages of examination, that is, after the history taking, the examination by palpation, palpatory examination and examination by movements, the therapist should be able to make an assessment of the patient's musculoskeletal condition and begin to put together a treatment plan for that patient.

Massage of the Neck and Shoulders

Massage of the neck and shoulders may be performed with the patient seated or lying on the treatment table. Seated massage of the neck and shoulders can be taught to give students a procedure they can follow easily and practise at home on

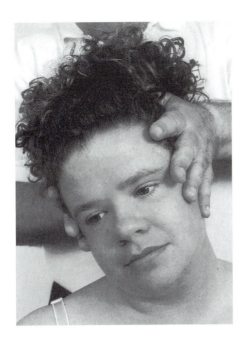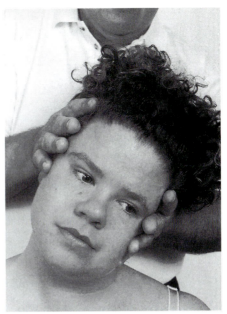

▲ *Figure 58*
(a) Resisted side bending to the right and; (b) resisted side bending to the left of the neck.

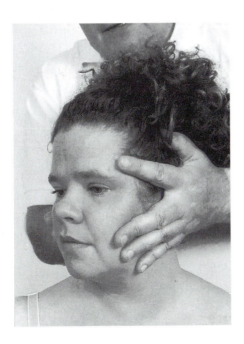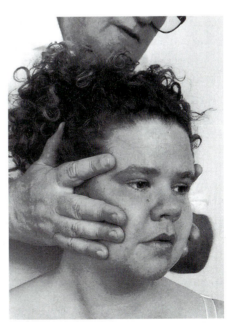

▲ *Figure 59*
(a) Resisted side turning to the right and; (b) resisted side turning to the left of the neck.

family or friends without having to rush out and acquire a treatment table. It gives them a little time before having to commit themselves to the expensive purchase of equipment.

The massage treatment starts with effleurage from the occiput down towards the upper thoracic spine. The pressure is on the downward sweep and eases as the hands return over the scapulae and shoulders and up the cervical spine. The downward pressure is in the same direction as the flow of the venous blood and the main lymphatic drainage.

Effleurage is followed by circular friction on either side of the spinous processes from a level at the top of the scapulae upward to the occiput. These circular frictions act upon the muscles and also provoke movement in different directions at each vertebral segment.

The petrissage movements concentrate initially upon the bulk of the trapezius muscle and involve lifting the muscle, lifting and squeezing the muscle, rolling the muscle anteriorly and posteriorly and wringing the muscle.

The therapist should now pay particular attention to the muscles around the medial scapulae. By placing the patient's arm behind them (sometimes this is not possible) the scapula is made to stand out posteriorly, allowing the therapist much better access to the muscles attaching from the scapula to the spine. This area is frictioned first one side then the other.

Deep, circular friction movements are also applied firmly to the accessible areas, anterior and posterior, of the glenohumeral joint.

Between each of the movements of massage, the therapist returns to effleurage of the area under treatment to stimulate the flow of blood and encourage the drainage from the tissues.

The therapist will perform hacking and clapping movements of tapotement if the intention is to tone and stimulate but often in treatment of conditions this aspect of massage is omitted and the patient is left in a very relaxed state.

Treatment of the Shoulder by Movements

Upon the completion of the massage, the remedial therapist will introduce some passive movement into the treatment. There are four therapeutic movements that can be used to excellent effect. The four movements should only be applied after the massage part of the treatment has been completed:

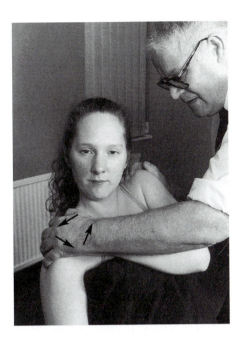

◄ *Figure 60*
Hand position for passive
shoulder circling movement.

1.   The patient sits and the therapist faces the patient. The patient places the
      hand of the injured shoulder across his chest diagonally and gently grasps his
      own opposite shoulder. The therapist places one hand on the patient's arm
      which is resting on the shoulder. The therapist's free hand then grasps the
      injured shoulder and passively circumducts the shoulder, first medially several
      times and then laterally several times.

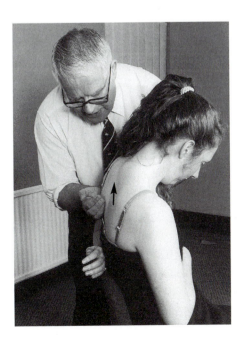

◄ *Figure 61*
Hand position for scapula lifting.

2. The patient sits and holds the arm on the affected side behind his back. He may flex his elbow and tuck the arm behind him on the chair. The therapist stands at the side of the patient and with his front hand he holds the head of the humerus in his hand and the rear hand holds the scapula from underneath. Both hands move together to lift the scapula, hold it briefly and then allow it to slide back into the starting position. This may be performed half a dozen or even more times and 'frees' the scapula from any adhesions that may be holding it to the thoracic cage.

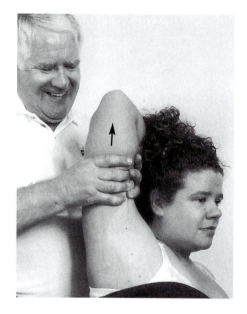

▶ *Figure 62*
Traction of the shoulder.

3. The third therapeutic movement is a shoulder traction. Again the patient is seated and the therapist stands at the side of the patient's affected shoulder. The therapist bends the patient's elbow and then grasps around the patient's biceps and triceps muscles. The bent arm is gently but steadily moved so that the elbow travels and points up towards the ceiling – or as near to that position as the patient can comfortably manage. At this point the therapist asks the patient to inhale deeply and then exhale. As the patient breathes out the therapist can lift the arm in the direction of the ceiling to apply a traction that he holds for twenty seconds.

4. The fourth therapeutic movement is performed again with the patient in the sitting position. A small towel is rolled and placed in the axilla on the affected side between the patient's arm and rib cage. The therapist places one hand on the top of the shoulder and applies a downward pressure. The therapist's other hand grasps the patient at the elbow of the affected side and, using the towel as a pivot, moves the patient's arm medially across the front of the chest.

Treatment of the Neck by Movements

Passive movements of the neck are performed after the massage treatment has been largely completed. They may be done with the patient seated or with the patient lying on his back on the treatment table. A little modification may be required and this will be dealt with in due course.

Examination in the Sitting Position

The patient's neck is moved into flexion and then extension several times by the therapist. The movements are very similar to the passive movements employed in the examination procedure of the neck. The movements of passive side bending and then passive side turning follow. Each is done several times slowly and to the point of the patient's tolerance.

Examination with the Patient Lying on the Table

The movements of passive flexion of the patient's neck are easily performed. These are followed by the movements of passive side bending and passive side turning. Each movement is performed firmly and with care; the patient must be monitored for any discomfort or pain.

By placing one hand into the tunnel created by the patient's head and the pillow, the therapist can induce an anterior-posterior movement of the cervical vertebrae which is performed several times. This is accomplished by placing a finger on a spinous process and pushing anteriorly before releasing the pressure.

A gentle but firm passive gliding action can also be done by the therapist by adjusting the position of his hands on the sides of the patient's head and moving the head steadily first to the left and then to the right and adjusting a hand to resist each movement a little. This is not a movement to be learned from the pages of a book but should be demonstrated a number of times to the student/practitioner who should then be allowed time to practise the movement under a tutor's supervision.

The levator scapulae muscles may benefit by being stretched by the therapist. The patient's head is cradled by the hand on the same side as the affected muscle. The other arm is placed behind the head and rests on the shoulder of the affected levator scapula. The hand supporting the patient's head is rested on the other forearm. Now lift the patient's head into flexion with the forearm and turn the head to the opposite shoulder with your hand. Keep contact with the forearm and back of the hand during this movement. Hold for fifteen seconds and release the hold in the reverse order.

Neck Traction

Neck traction may be applied manually after massage and passive movements. Due consideration must be given to any contra-indications for passive movements and traction of the neck and these should have already emerged during the examination procedure.

Have the patient lying upon the table on his back and the therapist standing at the top of the table behind the patient's head. Ensure that the patient is lying straight from feet to head and if necessary make any adjustments to achieve this end before applying the traction movement.

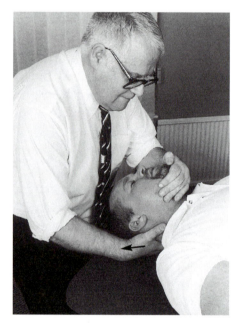

▶ *Figure 63*
Hand positions for neck traction.

The therapist takes a firm grasp of the patient's occiput in the palm of his hand. The other hand holds the patient under the chin without obstructing or putting pressure on the windpipe. If at all possible the therapist should brace his feet against the table legs as he begins this movement. (Some old illustrations show rather alarming methods of traction involving assistants pulling the therapist as he tractions the patient to achieve more pull).

Again the patient's breathing pattern can be usefully employed to facilitate the traction movement. Instruct the patient to breathe in deeply and then to exhale. As the patient breathes out the therapist eases his body backwards and maintains his hold on the occiput and lightly on the patient's jaw thus tractioning the neck.

This should be a smooth continuous movement and then the traction is held for fifteen to twenty seconds.

A neck traction may also be carried out on a seated patient. The therapist's hands are placed in the same position as for passive examination of the neck. The therapist should now flex his knees.

The neck is now taken into full extension and traction applied by pushing upwards with the thumbs aided by the effects of the therapist's body weight as the knees are simultaneously straightened.

Hand, Wrist, Elbow and Arm

Treatment records from a busy clinic will show varying incidence of treatments for arm conditions. These will include problems and injuries to the hand, the wrist and the elbow. However patients may present with conditions which show symptoms in the arm and have their origins elsewhere in the body. In some clinics these account for less than five per cent of all treatments. Mostly, patients visiting my clinic with arm problems tended to be people with overuse symptoms and pain around the elbow, for instance:

- Electricians.
- Heating engineers.
- Plumbers.
- Clerical and administrative workers.

In sport, there were representatives from:

- Skiing.
- Archery.
- All racquet sports.
- Croquet and, on one occasion, an aspiring professional darts player.
- Rock climbers, especially if they also fitted into one of the other categories are very vulnerable to elbow injuries.
- Golf.

A third group comprised of musicians; keyboard players and stringed instrument players to the fore. At one time my practice was very busy each year with a surge of music students. Many experienced quite severe problems by mid-term every Autumn due to the increase of intensity of playing much more frequently each day than they had played before starting their courses at the college.

The patients who experienced these activity-related injuries were usually found to be suffering from overuse and repetitive injuries. These were related either to hard, continuous gripping and/or unusual and intensive repetitive movements.

Examination of the Patient

When a patient comes to the treatment room with a problem concerning the arm, a full examination must be made of the patient as we have outlined in this book previously. This includes a visual examination of the patient in which the therapist must be able to see the patient from front, sides and back and must be able to visually examine both arms and shoulders. In other words, the patient must be suitably undressed and towelled for the examination.

Hand

The hand is the means of contact with the outside world, taken for granted until injury, loss of function or deformity occurs and the loss is quickly noticed and bitterly resented by the patient.

The patient will complain of various symptoms. These include pain, usually in the finger joints, the palm of the hand, or as a more generalised ache which may be referred from the neck or shoulder. There may be a deformity, perhaps of sudden appearance that may be a tendon injury or the more slowly appearing deformity of a bone or joint pathology.

Swellings may be localised or occur in several joints simultaneously. Loss of function may be reported as the patient having difficulty with eating or holding a glass, grasping objects, dressing or, quite distressingly, of difficulties with personal hygiene.

A patient displaying any unusual symptoms connected with the hand, including severe pain and tremor, should be referred quickly and without fuss to their GP for further investigation.

Look at both upper limbs and examine the patient for scars, unusual colouring of the skin, rough or smooth skin, dry or moist areas, muscle wasting, deformity, lumps and swellings. The hand is one of the more common sites of congenital deformity and the patient may have one of these:

1.   Total or partial absence of some part of the hand.
2.   Failure of differentiation, for example fingers joined together.
3.   Focal defects, for example an extra finger.

4. Overgrowth, for example a giant thumb.
5. Generalised malformation, for example Marfan's Syndrome.

Other patients may have an acquired deformity due to disorders of the skin, muscle and tendon injuries and joint conditions. Some cuts and severe burns are liable to heal with contracture of the skin. Arthritis may leave very visible signs of damage in the finger joints.

Infections of the hand are usually limited to one of several well-defined compartments and these include: paronychia, whitlows, infections from blisters, inflammation of tendon sheaths, and sudden and painful ballooning of the palm caused by a staphylococcus which has been implanted by a trivial or unobserved incident.

Continue the examination by palpating both hands and feeling for changes in temperature and texture of the skin, feel for nodules, swellings, thickenings in subcutaneous tissues and try and localise tenderness in any of the structures.

Examine the active movements of the fingers, for example curling the fingers into flexion and not only checking the range of movement but that all the fingers move. As far as possible request the patient to demonstrate movement at each joint individually. The patient should perform movement of the thumb in abduction from the hand both laterally and up towards the ceiling. The grip test is useful and this may be done by simply shaking both hands with the patient.

Examination of the Wrist

For the purpose of examination of the wrist the patient should expose both upper limbs to the therapist. The therapist should look for any scars, bruising, deformities, generalised or local swellings and he should compare the size of one forearm against the other.

This is followed by palpation in which the therapist feels for any undue changes or differences in temperature, searches for areas of tenderness and traces around the joints and bony landmarks of the wrist comparing size and shape.

The strength of the patient's grip of both hands should be assessed. The patient should be asked to place the palms of the hands together and then to elevate the elbows into the movement of dorsiflexion. Palmar flexion can be performed next, by placing the back of the hands together.

The movement of the hands medially and laterally, often described as radial and ulnar deviation may be done by asking the patient to tuck their elbows into their sides flexed at right angles and with the palms turned upwards. The patient is then requested to move the hands into the midline and then outwards away from the midline. The final movement to examine is that of pronation and supination, i.e. turning the palm of the hand down and then turning the palm upwards.

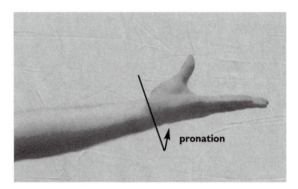

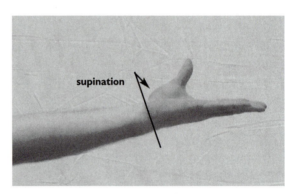

► *Figure 64*
(a) Pronation and;
(b) supination of the hand.

The therapist should ask the patient at the completion of each movement how the movement felt and should note the patient's range and ease of movement.

Examination of the Elbow

Symptoms of elbow conditions may include pain localised to the medial or lateral condyles of the humerus; pain arising in the joint is usually more diffuse. The patient may report that the joint is stiff or restricted in certain movements, for example unable to flex the elbow sufficiently to place food in the mouth, an inability to straighten the arm, or difficulty in carrying larger objects. Swelling around the joint may be due to an injury or inflammation. A lump right on the extremity of the elbow would suggest olecranon bursitis.

Tingling sensations in the hand may occur in an elbow disorder due to the proximity of the median nerve to the joint.

The therapist needs to examine both elbows with the upper limb suitably uncovered. Look at the patient as he stands with his arms held alongside the body and check each arm for valgus and varus. Wasting of muscles and sometimes lumps may be seen if the patient elevates both arms with the palms of the hands downwards.

The therapist palpates around the joint for warmth, tenderness, swelling and synovial thickening. Palpate the muscles to allow the elbow to function and, whilst palpating around the joint pay attention to the muscle attachments to the epicondyles. The head of radius can be palpated by gently pronating and supinating the forearm.

Each limb should be moved actively and then passively in flexion and extension and then, as for the wrist, in the movements of pronation and supination.

Nerve Supply to the Arm and Hand

The nerve supply to the arm is derived from the fourth cervical nerve to the first and second thoracic nerves. The three major nerves that supply the hand and arm are the median nerve, the ulnar nerve and the radial nerve.

Injury to any of these nerves, for example as the result of a fracture of the humerus, a deep laceration at the wrist or even sustained pressure in the axilla, may produce loss of function in some part or even a clawing of the fingers. These types of injury are the province of the medical consultant in the first place and massage therapists may be requested to work with such patients at the request or with the approval of the consultant.

On occasions, a patient may experience symptoms in the shoulder, arm and hand of a musculoskeletal nature that arise in the spine and cause a compression on the nerve root in the upper thoracic or lower cervical area. If this is suspected, the therapist should carry out an examination of the patient's back and neck and, if the cause of the symptoms is found, a treatment plan may be formulated.

Massage of the Hand and Arm

Sometimes patients experience stiffness and limitation of movement at the wrist after fracture, the popular one being the Colle's fracture. This is usually caused by a fall in which the hand tries to take the weight of the body and the fracture occurs at the distal radius and ulna that are also displaced backwards. Damage may also occur at the ulnar side of the wrist to both cartilaginous and ligamentous tissue. It is also possible that the median nerve may be compressed against the shaft of the radius.

Recovery is, in most cases, straightforward. However, there may be some residual stiffness that is unacceptable and inconvenient to the patient. Occasionally, the fracture may be more complicated and the patient may be left with some pain, stiffness and an inability to pronate and supinate the forearm; other movements may also be affected and muscles may have atrophied.

The treatment of the patient with post-Colle's fracture and after removal of the plaster cast, begins with a full, thorough and deep massage of the whole arm from hand to shoulder. Included in the massage are deep frictions at the elbow and around the wrist joints. The use of a faradic muscle stimulator for 2–3 minutes is often beneficial especially to the patients with the more complicated symptoms.

This should be followed by a series of passive movements performed by the therapist on the patient's wrist. The therapist grips the patient's forearm on the affected side securely with his left hand. He then grips the patient's hand in what is often described as a 'butcher's hook' grip and applies a traction to the wrist. Whilst maintaining the traction, the wrist is taken through its range of movements by the therapist, that is, into palmar flexion and dorsiflexion, ulnar and radial deviation, circumduction and pronation and supination.

After completing these passive movements several times the therapist now grips the distal ulna and radial heads and moves the heads up and down in opposite directions; 'shaking' the joint. The treatment is completed by effleurage of the whole limb.

Carpal Tunnel Syndrome

The patient complains of aching, pain and numbness in the distribution of the median nerve, worse at night, more often in females and may be aggravated by certain activities like knitting or even holding a newspaper. On examination direct pressure on the tunnel itself hurts the patient, as does palmar flexion against resistance.

This patient is probably suffering from carpal tunnel syndrome or compression of the median nerve at the flexor retinaculum, the small fibrous bridge that spans the small bones at the palm of the hand.

Sometimes this injury happens with sports men and women. There have been reports, for example, of incidence, of carpal tunnel syndrome amongst rowers at championship events where the intensity and frequency of competition and practise exceed the fitness levels of many of the participants and they are victims of this syndrome.

The flexor tendons, in their synovial sheaths, pass through the tunnel as does the median nerve which carries fibres to the muscles of the ball of the thumb, the index, middle and ring fingers. Pressure causes pain and/or tingling in these areas and feelings of weakness especially in the thumb. The balance of blood flow, innervation and lymphatic drainage is disturbed and may lead to ischaemia, loss of nutrient and build up of toxic waste in the area.   Adhesions may form in which the flexor tendons may adhere to their synovial sheaths and the separate sheaths may stick together and even though movement may be possible the movement causes pain.

Treatment of patients with carpal tunnel syndrome follows the procedure of a thorough massage to the whole limb. Frictions around the wrist may be introduced when the patient reports that the pain level has been reduced and the patient feels able to tolerate the friction movements.

Cold applications are useful in the early stages of treatment. It is perhaps a better use of time if the patient is instructed in the use of cold packs and applies them at home two or three times each day for up to fifteen minutes. The cold applications will help reduce inflammation and are also analgesic. Care must be taken to instruct the patient not use ice or cold packs from the freezer directly on the skin.

Some therapists use heat on their patients from the beginning of treatment rather than cold, feeling that this reduces the chances of adhesions forming.

For those therapists qualified in the use of electrotherapy, pulsed ultrasound with the setting at 0.5 for 3 minutes at first, rising to 5 minutes as the treatment progresses, is beneficial in most cases. Other conditions of the hand that can be helped to some degree by massage and movements include:

1.   Deputrens' contracture.
2.   Raynaud's disease.
3.   Osteoarthritis (which seldom attacks wrist
      or elbow but certainly affects fingers).
4.   De Quervain's disease.

Fracture of the scaphoid is often not diagnosed immediately and the therapist can help by being aware of this when a patient presents with a 'sprained wrist'. The fracture may be caused by a fall on to the outstretched hand with the wrist dorsiflexed or by the hand being struck by a hard object. The patient complains of pain at the base of the thumb and the radial aspect of the wrist that intensifies on movement. Pain is felt immediately on palpation dorsally of the patient's wrist distal to the radial styloid. The patient's grip is impaired. This patient should be referred to a GP or hospital for further examination and treatment.

Tenosynovitis and Lateral Epicondylitis

These painful conditions are found in the forearms of people who do a lot of sustained gripping in their everyday activities, for example, mechanics, electricians, even massage therapists.

The tendon glides through sheathing which contains a synovial membrane and this membrane may become inflamed and swollen. Sometimes it is possible to hear the noise, crepitus, if the therapist grasps the patient's forearm and asks the patient to clench his fist and then flex and extend the wrist. Massage over the painful area is not advised for this patient as it will aggravate rather than heal.

A condition that has some connection with tenosynovitis is lateral epicondylitis, also known as common extensor tendinitis or 'tennis elbow'. It is a common source of elbow pain in musicians, athletes, electricians, climbers and others who are required to sustain gripping actions. For example, use of a screwdriver or a racquet, or those required to suffer prolonged repetitive use of the forearm muscles, for example a repetitive action on an assembly line at work.

The patient history usually demonstrates that the injury is the result of demands made on the tissues that exceed the strength, endurance or flexibility of the wrist extensor muscles and tendons. Less commonly the condition may be the result of a single acute injury.

Many tennis, badminton and squash players are affected. Gripping a racquet, especially if this is allied to impact, for example hitting a ball and eccentric loading, for example a mis-hit backhand shot, can have serious effects on the player's forearm muscles. Other factors that may contribute include:

* Gripping too tightly.
* Unsuitable grip size.
* Excessive string tension.
* Excessive racquet weight.
* Faulty backhand technique.
* Putting top-spin on backhand shots.
* Hitting the ball off-centre.

The damage may not only be to the muscle tissue but also to the periosteal surface where the muscles attach to the bone.

With the overuse type of injury there is often a characteristic onset and progression of symptoms; perhaps a new racquet, a different technique or intensive playing. The early symptoms are probably feelings of fatigue in the arm and tightness in the muscles, followed by aching in the region of the lateral elbow. This may be followed by a sudden sharp pain during activity – especially on backhand shots or mis-hits. The pain eventually becomes constant and increases in severity. Play or activity becomes impossible and some daily activities become increasingly difficult to perform, for example carrying a bag, wringing out a cloth, even holding a cup of tea.

On examination there will be pain over or just distal to the lateral epicondyle of the humerus. There may also be pain in the muscles of the dorsum of the forearm, pain on active and certainly on resisted wrist extension and probably pain is experienced on passive wrist flexion. Atrophy and weakness of the forearm muscles will occur in chronic conditions.

The treatment of this condition is firstly by following the R.I.C.E.S. regime to allow the condition to begin healing. Rest from activities that aggravate and cause pain may be quite difficult to establish, especially if the rest means that the patient may have to stop work for an unspecified period of time. This is made worse if the patient is self-employed. The condition of the patient will deteriorate until the patient is forced to stop the aggravating activities but much more damage has occurred in the meantime. There have been reports in the press over the last two or three years which describe the very severe long-term effects of these injuries to people involved in compensation claims against employers in the courts.

The treatment in the chronic stages is by massage of the whole limb and frictions at the attachments into the humerus. The action of the frictions may hurt the patient and should be quite deep but of short duration, say five seconds.

The tissues may be stretched by a soft tissue manipulation in which the forearm is rapidly extended from the flexed position with the forearm pronated, the wrist plantar flexed and the fingers fully flexed.

Treatment by faradic muscle stimulation at each treatment session is beneficial and pulsed ultrasound helps most patients. I have used a Japanese machine called *Likon* on occasions and found it to be efficacious in treating this condition.

The introduction of gentle active exercise is part of the treatment. Many therapists combine the use of *Theraband* and heat treatment, keeping a careful watch for any adverse reaction.

There is a choice of proprietory pads and supports for the treatment and prevention of this condition. You may fashion such a pad from chiropody felt and, after flexing the elbow to ninety degrees, place the pad about one inch down from the crease made by the movement of flexion and secure it with non-stretch tape.

Rehabilitation aims to restore the strength, endurance and flexibility of the wrist extensor muscles. The patient must be informed that exercise may worsen the condition if done too vigorously or too soon. The period of rest should be until the patient can perform mild exercise without pain and without painful after-effects. A combination of fast contraction and light resistance exercises with *Theraband* are usually well tolerated and muscular endurance may be built up steadily but gently.

The patient must not resume the activities that caused the condition until the treatment is concluded. A good test for the patient is can they perform resisted dorsiflexion of the wrist without experiencing any pain. Technique changes in the way the patient performs the activities should also form part of the overall treatment plan.

Olecranon Bursitis

Olecranon bursitis used to be known in lay terms as 'Student's Elbow' or 'Miner's Elbow' and referred to the swelling of the bursa on the very end of the elbow. Bleeding into the bursa causes inflammation and swelling.

The causes may be repetitive pressure and friction, as in coal mining. I recollect from my time as a wrestler that many of us suffered olecranon bursitis periodically and the egg-like bumps protruding from elbows were known as 'wrestler's friends'. The consensus was that it was caused by constantly banging our arms on the canvas, for example during a break-fall.

Direct trauma can cause acute haemorrhagic bursitis and turf burns and lacerations from a fall or accident can lead to septic bursitis.

The symptoms of olecranon bursitis are swelling, variable pain and tenderness, limitation of flexion at the elbow. There may be discolouration. On further examination, pressure over the centre of the bursa brings the edges into sharp definition.

The condition is treated by rest from aggravating activities, cold treatments and compression by tubigrip bandage or neoprene sleeve, for at least the first two days. It is a good idea to look for the cause of the bursitis and take preventative measures for the future that may include the wearing of a pad to protect the elbow.

Back

Patients with back pain are perhaps the biggest single group requesting treatment from a massage therapist. It is not uncommon to spend a full day in the treatment room and treat only patients with back pain.

Back pain is a common scourge that affects the majority of the population of the UK at some time in their lifetime. More than 11 million working days are lost in the UK, costing British industry five billion pounds (Carter, 2000). Four out of five workers suffer from back pain and 20% take time off work because of it (Unison Survey, 2000).

The pain may occur anywhere in the back, for example, a pain between the shoulder blades or a painful tightness around the waist but pain in the lumbar area is the most common. In spite of increasing mechanisation and computerisation, shorter working hours and the advances in medical science, the incidence of back pain does not seem to decrease.

Structure and Tissues

The spine is a flexible column formed by a series of bones called vertebrae. In between the vertebrae are cartilaginous cushions called discs. The vertebrae are held in position by a series of ligaments. Movement of the spine is from the muscles of the back.

Vertebrae

In an adult there are 33 individual vertebrae. They are divided into groups:

1. 7 Cervical.
2. 12 Thoracic.
3. 5 Lumbar.
4. 1 Sacral (5 fused vertebrae).
5. 1 Coccygeal (4 fused vertebrae).

The vertebrae stand one on top of the other and form a strong pillar to support the head and trunk. They form a hollow cylinder behind their bodies to contain and protect the spinal cord and they help the body through its wide range of movements. Each vertebra consists of two main parts:

1. Anterior segment or body.
2. Posterior segment or neural arch.

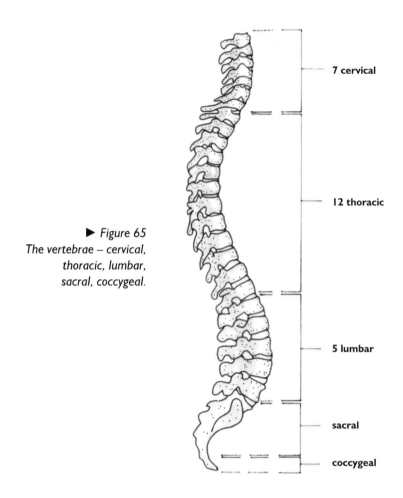

▶ *Figure 65*
The vertebrae – cervical,
thoracic, lumbar,
sacral, coccygeal.

7 cervical

12 thoracic

5 lumbar

sacral

coccygeal

The cervical vertebrae are smaller than those of the thoracic and lumbar regions and the first and second, known as Atlas (C1) and Axis (C2) are designed to allow nodding and rotary movements. There are no cushioning discs between Atlas and the skull and between Atlas and Axis. C1 is difficult to palpate in most people and is perhaps best felt in a relaxed neck between the angle of the jaw and the occiput when side turning the head.

The second vertebra (C2) has a larger spinous process and is usually the first vertebra to be palpated when working from the skull towards the shoulders.

The seventh cervical vertebra has a longer spinous process which can be easily seen and palpated in most people and is known as vertebra prominens.

The thoracic area of the spine is the largest and perhaps least mobile section. The vertebrae are intermediate in size compared to the smaller cervical vertebrae and the larger lumbar vertebrae. Present on the sides of the bodies of the thoracic vertebrae are facets and demi-facets for the articulation of the heads of the ribs.

The lumbar vertebrae are the largest of the vertebrae and articulate with the sacrum, a large triangular bone inserted like a wedge between the innominate bones of the hip. The sacrum curves posteriorly and forms the attachment for many of the important muscles of the spine.

In the majority of people a line from both iliac crests will take the hands of the therapists to the disc between L4 and L5 vertebrae. L4 spinous process is comparatively large and may be mistaken for the deeper and blunter L5 vertebra. At the end of the spine is the coccyx that may fuse with the sacrum in later life.

Spinal Cord

The spinal cord is a continuation from the brain and is cylindrical. It is some 42–45cms in length and occupies the spinal canal from Atlas (C1) to the first Lumbar vertebra (L1) where it continues by slender filaments or strands.

There are 31 spinal nerves that take their origin from the spinal cord and are transmitted through the intervertebral foramina on either side of the spinal column.

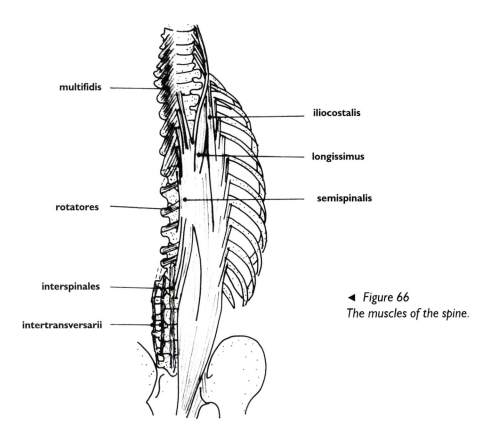

multifidis

iliocostalis

longissimus

semispinalis

rotatores

interspinales

intertransversarii

◀ *Figure 66*
The muscles of the spine.

Muscles of the Spine

The muscles of the spine may be grouped in several different ways, for example into:

1. Long muscles that pass at least 7 vertebrae, e.g. iliocostalis, longissimus.
2. Average back muscles that pass between 2 and 6 vertebrae, e.g. semispinalis, multifidis.
3. Short back muscles that go to the nearest vertebra, e.g. rotatores, interspinales, intertransversarii.

All the muscles of the back work together to produce movement and also work in collaboration with the abdominal muscles which, when strong can have a very helpful role, or, when weak can add to the strain upon the spinal muscles.

The longer muscles, the erector spinae have origins and insertions from the sacrum, the lumbar vertebrae and the iliac crest and attach into ribs, thoracic and cervical vertebrae and into the skull.

Movements of the Spine

Flexion is the most extensive movement of the spinal column. There is more flexion in the lumbar spine than the cervical.

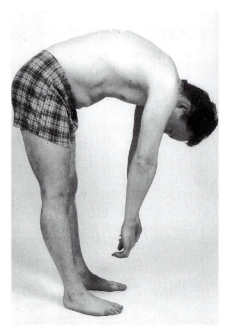 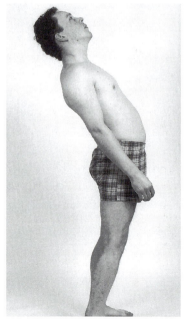

▲ *Figure 67*
(a) Standing flexion and; (b) standing extension of the spine.

Less extensive is the movement of extension which is limited by the anterior longitudinal ligament and the closeness of the spinous processes. There is more extension in the cervical spine than in the lumbar.

Lateral flexion or side bending, is limited by spinal ligaments and the closeness of the transverse processes.

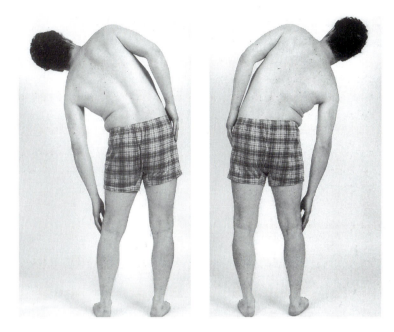

▲ *Figure 68*
(a) Standing side bend to the left and; (b) standing side bend to the right of the spine.

Rotation or twisting is the combined effects of small movements at each segment, each contributing to a larger movement when the whole spine is involved. Some circumduction is possible and is produced by a succession of the other movements.

The cervical area enjoys the greatest freedom of movement. The thoracic area is much more limited, with the exception of rotation or twisting and the lumbar area is free in flexion, has extension and lateral movement but no rotation. The vertebrae can move in some or all of the following different ways:

1. Distraction/compression.
2. Anterior/posterior.
3. Laterally.
4. Flexion/extension.
5. Side bending.
6. Rotation.

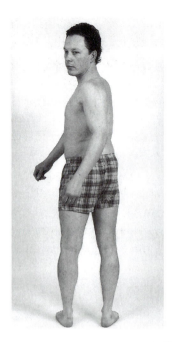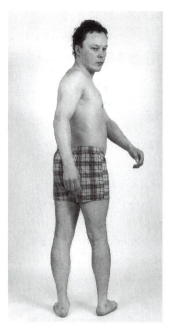

▲ *Figure 69*

(a) Standing rotation to the left and; (b) standing rotation to the right of the spine.

Spinal Ligaments

The anterior longitudinal ligament is a broad and strong band of fibres which extends along the anterior surfaces of the vertebral bodies from axis to sacrum and blend with and reinforce the discs.

The posterior longitudinal ligament is situated within the spinal canal from axis to sacrum and also blends with and reinforces the discs.

The ligamentum flavum is more elastic and connects the laminae, the posterior segments of the vertebrae. It is not present between occiput and atlas and atlas and axis.

Smaller ligaments also have a role to play and these include those connecting the articular processes, the capsular ligaments and those connecting the spinous processes, the supraspinous, interspinous and intertransversarii ligaments.

Causes of Back Pain

1. General diseases in which back pain can occur, for example influenza or other viral infections.
2. Pain referred to the back from visceral diseases, e.g. pleurisy, kidney disease.

3.   Diseases of the vertebral column and nervous system, e.g. osteoarthritis, neoplasm. Osteoarthritis may occur in the spinal joints and it may occur elsewhere in the body and disturb posture thus affecting the spine. Arthritis limits movement at joints and thus muscles and other tissues and structures cannot perform normally. With the passage of time, changes occur in these tissues and structures. Spinal balance may become upset and areas of the spine put under constant strain so that a sudden wrench or fall, for example, will lead to immediate injury.

4.   Muscular injuries are perhaps the most common cause of back pain. A strained muscle loses the power of regulating its circulation efficiently and waste products remain in the fibres. The muscle becomes overloaded and becomes aching and painful and prone to further injury. Muscles may be injured by repetitive movements, poor posture or by single traumatic incidents. The first mild sunny weekend in early spring usually meant a procession of back pain patients during the following week. Many were in severe pain due to muscle strain, leading to painful spasm caused by venturing out into the garden to dig and hoe, pull and push and all the other vigorous garden activities. This after several months relative inactivity followed by a sudden and sustained bout of heavy work.

5.   Back pain caused by mechanical faults, e.g. scoliosis, kyphosis, intervertebral disc lesion.

6.   The unavoidable processes of ageing and degeneration on the tissues and structures of the back.

With age the whole spine tends to stiffen, the total range of movements reduces and the shock absorbing capacity lessens. Ageing affects everyone and it is often the combined effects of ageing with other conditions that is critical, for example the combination of ageing and health or ageing and lifestyle.

Degeneration may start during the late teenage years and it may begin in one particular disc, joint or ligament only. Degeneration tends to begin earlier in those who do heavy work or violent sport and the accompanying training. It is more likely to be the result of hard but unskilled effort or poor technique. It usually starts as minor damage to discs, vertebral bodies or ligaments. The cumulative effects of repeated damage that may go virtually unnoticed at the time are thought to be very significant.

Discs become thinner, flatter, stiffer and more fibrous. The nucleus dries out and the load bearing capability decreases. Ligaments become less efficient and begin to have a more restrictive effect on joints. Articulating facet cartilages suffer damage and do not offer the previous level of protection. Osteophytes may form around processes and on facets due to trauma.

The overall effects of ageing and degeneration is discomfort and pain, loss of function to some degree and this will vary from person to person depending upon other factors.

For some time it has been suspected that driving and the effects of vibration from machinery causes back pain. The Health and Safety Executive published a leaflet (1999) which pointed at the mounting evidence that drivers of some types of industrial vehicles suffer back pain earlier than other workers and that some of them will leave their work at a comparatively young age because of it. Among those at most risk were drivers of:

1. Construction and quarrying vehicles and machinery;
2. Tractors and other agricultural and forestry machinery;
3. Industrial trucks such as forklift trucks and straddle carriers;
4. Road haulage vehicles, rail vehicles, buses, etc.

Back damage can be caused by vibration passing through the seat into the driver's body through the buttocks and is known as 'whole body vibration'. Those operating large static compaction, hammering or punching machinery can also be exposed to high levels of vibration that pass from the platform of the machine into the operator via the feet.

Not only are industrial drivers at risk. An article in the *American Journal of Epidemiology* (1975) stated that driving either causes back pain or contributes to it. Brian McIlwraith, osteopath, has long lectured and written about the ill-effects many drivers suffer from poor seat and pedal positioning and the effects of vibration and acceleration/deceleration and pointed out the low priority placed by manufacturers and buyers on back health. Disc players, alloys, leather seats, power steering and the rest, head the queue in front of, say, a lumbar support.

There are other causes of back pain which do not fit quite so neatly into the categories mentioned above, for example, stress, tension, anxiety. Back pain is often experienced during pregnancy and can be linked to menstrual problems.

Any abnormal strain on a normal back may lead to injury. Normal daily stresses on a back that is abnormal may lead to pain and even normal stresses on a normal back which is unprepared for the stress can cause damage and pain.

Back Examination

As in any other condition, a thorough examination of the patient is required before attempting to plan any massage treatment. A full medical history must be taken from the patient together with a full account of the onset and progress of the presenting condition.

The therapist carries out an on-going visual examination of the patient from the moment of first contact and many indicators may be gained about the nature of the injury by watching the patient walk, sit down, get off a chair or remove his coat. Sometimes movement is obviously very difficult and the patient is in much pain.

On occasions I have been called out to patients experiencing severe back pain and unable to consider travelling to the treatment room. The patient may be in bed or may be covered by a duvet on the carpet in the room where the severe pain struck them down. Much useful information can be given by a spouse or partner and should be sought by the therapist, especially if the patient is in severe pain and unable to give much useful information.

The therapist on these occasions may be dealing with a patient with a herniated disc or with a condition outside of the therapist's experience or qualification and the therapist must be prepared to refer to the patient's GP or to the local hospital.

Signs and Symptoms

Pain is the predominant feature for most patients with back conditions and it is the principal reason why the patient seeks treatment. The onset of pain may be sudden, for example, after lifting a heavy object, or of gradual onset without any antecedent event. The pain may be constant or there may be periods of remission. The pain may be related to a particular posture or movement, for example, sitting down.

The patient may be a little vague in his description of the pain and where exactly the pain is felt. The pain may be variously described as:

1. Dull.
2. Burning.
3. Sharp.
4. Like toothache in my back.

The pain may not only be felt in the back but may travel into the buttocks, thigh and leg. This type of pain is often described as 'sciatica' and may indicate compression on one of the lumbar or sacral nerve roots. Sometimes patients may complain of tingling, 'pins and needles', even numbness in the affected limb. Among the possible causes for these symptoms are herniation of a disc, arthritic lipping and joint injury. Each patient must be examined thoroughly and this includes questions about the onset and nature of the pain they are experiencing.

Pain may be accompanied by what patients may describe as 'stiffness'. This may be sudden and complete as with a disc lesion. Stiffness may be continuous but with times of increasing severity and times of much lower concern, for example many patients complain of stiffness in their backs early in the morning and that the stiffness lessens as the day progresses. This may suggest arthritis or ankylosing spondylitis. One of my long-term patients told me that every day he experienced severe stiffness but on getting on his feet and becoming active the stiffness disappeared completely and his range of movement was excellent – until awakening next morning. X-ray investigation showed that osteoarthritis was well established in his lumbar spine.

The patient may have a deformity, for example a scoliosis, a lateral deviation or an excessive lordosis in the lumbar spine or an excessive lordosis in the thoracic spine. Another patient may present with a complete loss of the lumbar lordosis. Sometimes the deformity is of a long-standing origin, other times the deformity is temporary and brought on, for example, by a severe muscle spasm. Some patients with pain originating from an intervertebral disc may, for instance, stand and walk with their bodyweight held away from the side of the lesion.

Paraesthesia and numbness may be felt in the lower limbs but they can usually be related to one of the nerve pathways. If these symptoms are relieved by rest and sitting and then aggravated by standing and walking the patient may be displaying symptoms of spinal stenosis and should be referred to his GP for further action.

Examination of the Patient in a Standing Position

Watch how the patient walks, sits and undresses. The patient should undress to their underwear for this examination and the process of undressing should yield further clues to the therapist.

Check the static posture of the patient from the front, back and sides. Look for scars, unusual contours and creases in the skin, obvious deformity, general shape and posture, distribution of body weight, symmetry at all the major anatomical landmarks.

Visually and then manually check the arches of the patient's feet whilst in the standing position. Any podiatrist worth his salt will tell you unhesitatingly that a good proportion of back pain originates from fallen arches. Problems and injuries to the feet will have knock-on effects to other parts of the body (Seager, 2000).

The patient should now be asked to perform a series of movements. Inability or inhibition to perform should be noted. Check forward flexion but take care not to confuse stiffness in the hamstrings with stiffness in the spine. The hamstrings and lumbar-pelvic rhythm can be assessed by toe-touching with the knees straight. In flexion the smoothness of the curve of the spine from the lower cervical down to the sacrum should be observed. Flat areas may denote a loss of normal movement between vertebral bodies which adversely affect normal activity of nerves and circulation around the joints and neighbouring soft tissues. Such a fixation produces a constant pressure on the articulating surfaces, one on the other. This may cause an irritation to the nerve fibres supplying these surfaces and eventually disordered activity spreading to the spinal nerves and their roots. Keep a watchful eye on how much the patient employs hip flexion in this movement.

The patient is now asked to flex or bend sideways to the left and to the right with their arms by their sides. Compare the range of movement on each side and look for symmetrical curves during the movement. A loss of symmetry may indicate a fixation.

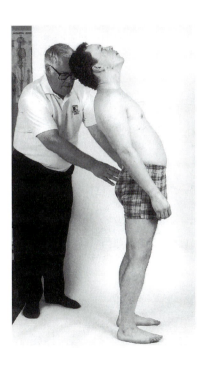

◄ *Figure 70*
Extension of the spine supervised and supported by the therapist.

The movement of extension follows and the patient is requested to extend backwards as far as possible. It is a good idea to stand near enough to offer support should the patient require it during this movement. The patient should keep their legs straight and not bend their knees. During extension the lumbar curve should be anterior and thoracic spine quite straight. If the lumbar curve is not anterior and the thoracic curve is more posterior than it should be in this movement it would indicate a fixation.

The movements of rotation may be assessed by asking the patient to hold their arms out at shoulder level and twist around to the left and right without moving the hip girdle. Discomfort and limitation on these movements would indicate a lumbar problem.

Rib movement during breathing can also be monitored during this examination. There should be a seven centimetre difference between inhalation and exhalation. Interference with normal breathing is one of the first effects of muscle spasm – the more severe the spasm the more the interference. Patients with sudden onset muscle spasm often report on how they had difficulty breathing or that they cannot take a deep breath because of the pain.

Examination of the Back by Palpation

The examination by palpation is better done with the patient lying prone on the table. All the spinous processes, including those away from the area of pain, should be palpated as well as the soft tissue either side of the spine for tender or painful areas, spasm or thermal changes.

Treatment of Back Pain

The massage therapist will employ several tools in the treatment of back pain, including rest, massage, thermal therapy, electrotherapy and movement/exercise. He will select his methods of treatment to suit the needs of each individual patient.

The great majority of back pain sufferers have pain, stiffness, loss of range of movement and various other symptoms as the result of muscle injury. A much smaller group has more serious problems such as disc herniation. The larger group, the patients with muscular problems will be discussed first and the patients with disc problems secondly.

Rest

In recent times the medical press has urged that rest as treatment for these muscular conditions be treated with some reservation in contrast to former times when rest appeared to be the treatment of choice for all back conditions.

Rest may mean the exclusion of activities that cause pain and aggravate the patient's condition rather than the concept of total rest in bed. The patient can continue with his normal activities whilst experiencing back pain and if these activities do not aggravate the pain this is the path to follow. Activity is, in most cases, preferable to inactivity; some kind of activity is better than none at all.

Inactivity over a period of just a few days has not only physical effects but may also have psychological effects that will hinder eventual recovery and return to work. Minor cases of back injury may be transformed into long-term problems by ceasing activity and becoming inactive. Activity, movement, exercise are all factors in the treatment of patients with back pain.

Massage

Back massage commences with the patient lying face down on the treatment table with back fully exposed but the rest of the body covered by towels to keep the patient warm and to keep the patient as secure and as relaxed as possible.

The first phase of the massage is effleurage from the sacrum and gluteal area with both hands, one on either side of the spinal column, up the body towards the head. The pressure of the effleurage is stronger on the upward stroke towards the head. At the completion of the upward stroke the therapist's hands travel laterally towards the shoulders and then lightly down to the start position at the sacrum. The pressure of each stroke is firm on the upward stroke and much lighter on the downward stroke.

Effleurage is followed by lateralising a sideways effleurage that helps take the tension out of 'tight' spinal muscles.

Frictioning of the spine is an arduous but necessary procedure and it is potentially dangerous to the therapist's thumbs. Many therapists damage their thumbs by incorrect technique when frictioning patient's backs. Some sustain severe damage and this will limit their activities as therapists and, sometimes, forces them to cease altogether.

An adjustable table is most helpful in limiting damage to a practitioner's thumbs when giving friction treatments. However, in the absence of an adjustable table there are other measures that may be taken to prevent injury to the therapist.

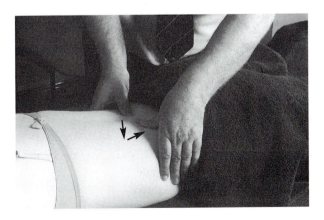

◄ *Figure 71*
Friction movement
of the spine.

The method for friction treatment to the patient's spine is to position the thumbs at the base of the patient's back just above the sacroiliac joint with the thumbs resting on the transverse processes of the lower lumbar spine, i.e. about 2–3 cms on either side of the spinous processes.

The therapist's thumbs rest on the muscles that lie above the transverse processes on either side of the spinous processes. The therapist should endeavour to stand close to the position of his thumbs as he begins to employ circular friction movements with both thumbs into the area of the lower lumbar spine.

The progression is up the spine towards the head with the thumbs continuing to give the deep firm friction at each level of the spine. The therapist must keep his head and body weight above his thumbs at all times. Thus, as he progresses up the spine to the thoracic and lower cervical area he makes sure that he moves his body alongside the table in the same direction as his hands.

The pressure through the thumbs and into the muscles and joints of the spine is derived from the therapist's body weight and not exclusively from the strength of the therapist's wrists and thumbs. The therapist should feel little fatigue and discomfort using this method. Get it wrong and the treatment becomes an ordeal for the therapist with the probability of long-term injury to the thumbs.

The friction treatments are most valuable in so far as they have a very beneficial effect upon the muscles, including the deeper layers of muscles, the spinal ligaments and the movement of the spinal joints themselves.

Further effleurage follows the frictions of the spine which may be performed two or three times depending upon the needs of the patient.

Petrissage movements are performed where appropriate, to accessible areas of latissimus dorsi, trapezius and levator scapulae.

Tapotement may be used if the overall effects of the treatment are to stimulate and energise the patient.

Treatment by Movements

After completion of the massage treatment the therapist may employ various movements to stretch and mobilise the patient's muscles and joints.

With the patient prone the therapist places his superior hand on the sacrum and the finger pads of the inferior hand on the ilium. He maintains a constant pressure on the sacrum and lifts and relaxes the ilium until some movement is felt.

The erector spinae muscles may be stretched by placing one hand over the sacrum and gently and continually rocking the patient from side to side whilst placing the back of the forearm across one side of the back. Count slowly to four while turning the forearm, hold the pressure again for a count of four and then slowly release for another count of four. The arm may now be placed in another position so that the whole of the back will be treated eventually, first one side of the spine and then the other. Continue with the steady rocking movement of the sacrum all the time whilst applying the gentle stretch.

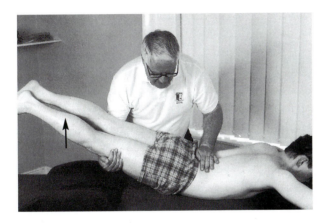

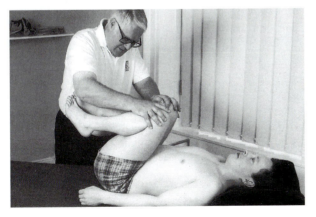

◄ *Figure 72*
(a) Passive extension and;
(b) passive flexion
of the spine.

Turn the patient on to their side facing you. Ask the patient to bring their knees up towards their chest and rest them against the therapist's thighs. The therapist leans over the patient and places the pads of his fingers between the spinous processes of the lumbar spine. Maintain pressure and gently rock from side to side until the soft tissue releases.

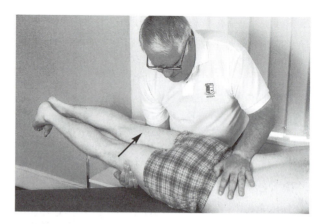

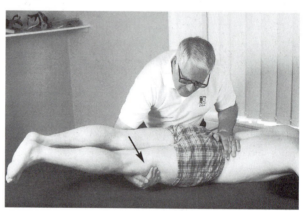

▶ Figure 73
(a) Passive side bend
to the left and;
(b) passive side bend
to the right of the spine.

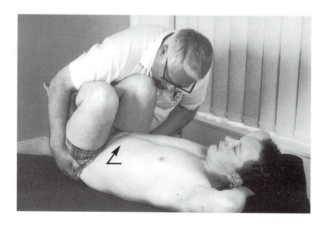

▶ Figure 74
Flexion side bending
of the spine.

Move the pads of the fingers onto the soft tissue, sustain the pressure into the muscles and continue rocking backwards and forwards until the muscles relax.

Now ask the patient to straighten the underneath leg and keep the upper leg in flexion. The therapist places his inferior hand over the lumbar spine and locks off the lower part of the body between his thigh and the inferior hand. The superior hand is placed on the front of the patient's upper shoulder which is then rolled away backwards from the therapist. The therapist maintains his hold on the lumbar spine and pulls it simultaneously towards him. The therapist holds the patient in this stretch position and then begins to gently work the spine by rocking it towards and then away.

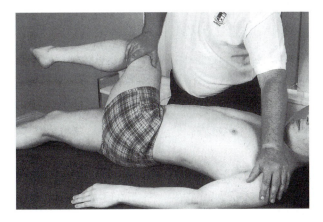

◀ *Figure 75*
Rotation of the spine.

With the patient in the supine position bring both knees up to the patient's chest and hold in this position which gives a stretch to the muscles of the spine.

The therapist may pinion the patient in this position by holding the knees down with his own chest and by holding either side of the table with his hands. Ask the patient to push up against the therapist's chest with both knees. Hold this position for seven seconds and then ask the patient to relax. The patient is then asked to inhale deeply and then exhale. On the out-breath move the knees even closer to the patient's chest and then to push again for seven seconds before relaxing. This may be done three times and the patient's lower back will be much more relaxed.

Intervertebral Disc Injury

Intervertebral discs are tough, fibro-elastic capsules made up of between 20–30 concentric layers and containing a colloidal gel in the middle. Each disc is basically a hydraulic shock absorber. The discs are avascular and receive nutrition via osmosis during periods of sleep and rest. There are no pain receptors in the disc and, of itself, does not cause pain. However, the pain felt by the patient from a disc injury can be of the most severe kind.

Degeneration of discs is common to all but the timing and rate of degeneration varies individually. Defects, injuries and degenerative changes may affect the whole spinal system and may produce severe pain and limitation of function.

Disc injury may be caused by; excessive forces, prolonged tension and poor posture, faulty annulus fibrous (outer wall), other pathologies and repeated minor trauma. There is a belief, common among therapists, that trauma sustained in early years may lie dormant and then combine with the appearance of the degenerative processes to produce a crisis.

Compression or pressure can cause a bulging of a disc and the outer wall may in turn put pressure on the posterior longitudinal ligament which in turn may allow pressure on a nerve root or its dural sheathing. This bulging of a disc wall may be caused by inadequate diet, poor work posture, 'flu, or degenerative processes. An example may be a middle-aged sedentary worker with poor sitting posture, lack of exercise and the degenerative processes well under way. Add to this a sudden, unaccustomed series of movements, e.g. the monthly shop at the local supermarket with firstly the risky experience of pushing a full trolley and, secondly, the action of transferring the various items from the trolley to the car boot. The twisting turning movements of unloading and reloading whilst bending over and transferring the weighty objects may put an unsustainable pressure on a disc.

In the worse possible cases the walls of the disc are so weakened that they burst open and the gel from the nucleus escapes through the fibrous capsule. The patients who suffer this extreme injury will immediately require the services and skills of a hospital.

Degeneration

Discs make up one third of the height of the vertebral column. Healthy discs are part of the functional integrity of the spine:

1. They separate the vertebral bodies, thus elongating the spine and keeping a substantial space between the vertebrae allowing the nerves to pass clearly from the spinal cord.
2. Along with the ligaments (especially the longitudinal ligaments and ligamentum flavum) exert the correct and balancing tensions necessary for spinal movement.
3. They maintain the correct functional distances for the facet joints.
4. They keep the foramina open.
5. They act as shock absorbers.

Degeneration is predictable and changes may occur as early as the late teens. Concentric tears may occur in the annular fibres. Radial tears from the centre outwards may happen. Degeneration tends to be worse on posterior and lateral segments of the discs. There may be an hereditary factor involved in disc injuries.

Some seventy-five per cent of disc degeneration occurs at the discs between L4 and L5 and L5 and the sacrum.

Disc Pressure

Disc pressure varies according to the position of the body and external stress.

- There is least pressure when the patient adopts the 'psoas position' because this reduces the pull of the iliopsoas muscles on the discs.
- Sitting produces greater pressure than standing.
- Younger bodies can generally tolerate twice the amount of pressure than older bodies.
- Weight carrying increases disc pressure and asymetrical loading, for example carrying a heavy suitcase, is even worse.
- Sustained pressure squeezes fluid out of the nucleus (this has been measured on weightlifters by sports scientists).
- Perhaps the worse stresses occur in simultaneously lifting and rotating, as in the monthly shop at the supermarket already referred to, when the pressure is on the posterior segment of the disc which is nearest to the sensitive tissues.
- Healthy abdominal and healthy back muscles help reduce disc pressure. Abdominal muscles help stabilise the spine. If the abdominal muscles are weak they cannot work effectively and strain is passed on to the back muscles and the iliopsoas muscles. In many cases abdominal exercises play a part in the treatment plan.

Symptoms

There will probably be a history of minor trauma with, perhaps, a more traumatic incident just before the onset of pain. The pain is usually back pain, variously described as aching, burning, dull, sharp, tender. The pain may refer across the lower back into the buttock(s), posterior or lateral thigh, calf, ankle and even to the toes. There may be a feeling of weakness in the legs.

The back pain is usually lumbar (the lumbar lordosis is lost) or sacral; sometimes across the back and sometimes one-sided. Acute muscle spasm is usually triggered in the muscles of the back. This contributes greatly to the pain already being felt by the pressure on the posterior longitudinal ligament and pressure on the dural sheath which refers the pain down the leg. Compression on the nerve root gives the numbness and weakness in the muscles.

Lateral flexion is limited and there is often lateral deviation away from the affected side. Activity aggravates the condition and in many cases proves to be very painful but the pain is relieved somewhat by rest.

Tests

There are a number of tests to find out if a patient has a disc problem. They include:

1. The Straight Leg Raising Test (Lasegue's Sign).
2. Drop Leg Test.
3. Leg Raise Sitting Test.
4. Cross Sciatic Straight Leg Raising Test (Fajersztaju's Sign).
5. The Charnley Test.
6. Foenig's Test.
7. Tests for upper lumbar disc injury.
8. L5 Disc Testing.

Perhaps the best known and most used procedure is the combination of the Straight Leg Raising Test (SLR) with the Drop Leg Test to give an indication of a disc lesion at the L4 and L5 level where most problems occur.

The patient lies on his back. The therapist begins to raise the patient's leg on the affected side, flexing the hip but keeping the knee in extension. From about thirty degrees a traction is applied to the sciatic nerve followed by a downward movement of the nerve roots in their foramina. The greatest movement occurs at

▶ *Figure 76*
Straight leg raising test
for L5-L4 disc injury.

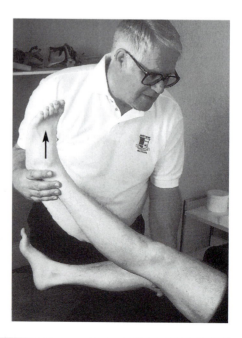

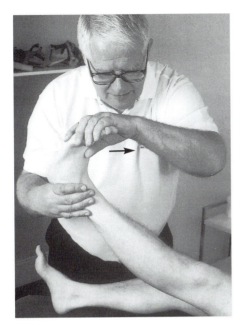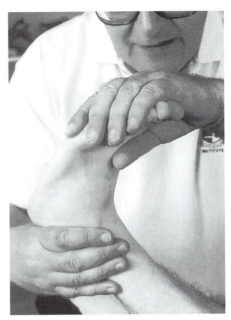

▲ *Figure 77*
Straight Leg Raising Test with dorsiflexion of the ankle.

L5, with some movement at L4 but no movement at the upper lumbar sites. The greatest degree of movement occurs when the leg is raised beyond sixty degrees. Thus, disc injury at L5 gives a strong reaction. (A negative SLR test does not rule out an upper lumbar disc injury).

A positive Straight Leg Raising Test is a good indicator of a disc lesion. The therapist may then lower the straight leg to within 5cms of the table and then let the leg drop the remaining distance. A positive reaction to this test combined with the previous test is a very strong indication of disc injury.

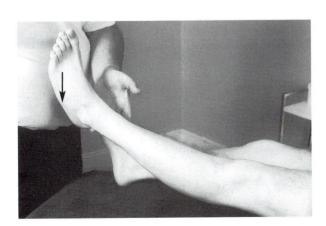

◀ *Figure 78*
Drop leg test
for disc injury.

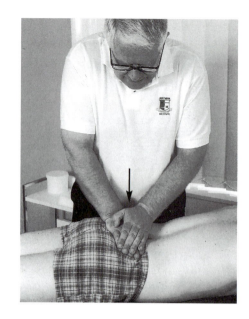

► *Figure 79*
Direct pressure over L5-L4
area to test for disc injury.

Other Signs of Disc Injury

Numbness replacing pain may indicate a more massive and prolonged pressure at the nerve root. Weakness and dysfunction of the hamstrings, gastrocnemius and gluteus maximus is also a strong indicator of an L5 disc injury.

Upon coughing and/or sneezing the patient experiences pain down the leg. This is suggestive of disc herniation but not conclusive on its own. Both actions require forceful contraction of the muscles and increase spinal fluid pressure which produces pain. There is often bowel and bladder dysfunction with L5 and L4 disc injury.

Problems at the upper lumbar discs refer their pain from posterior to anterior, to the area of the quadriceps which may also show weakness. The SLR Test is usually negative nor is there likely to be a bowel and/or bladder dysfunction. The knee jerk reflex is likely to be affected rather than the ankle jerk reflex involved in lower lumbar lesions.

Treatment of Disc Patients

My first concern is that the patient with a disc problem gets at least two days rest. Rest allows the disc to begin the process of natural healing in which it will receive nutrition and restoration of its shape. The patient must rest either lying on his back or in the psoas position. It may be that more than two days rest is required but this may be adjusted later. However, some movement should be encouraged at this time as prolonged rest will have bad effects on other tissues, particularly the spinal muscles (see stretching on page 168).

The emphasis should also be upon relaxation of the mind as well as the body. It is not a good idea to move the computer into the bedroom and then try to continue running the business from there. Relaxation enables the healing process to commence.

Some therapists encourage a detoxification diet followed by a light diet with extra Vitamin C and magnesium. Certainly alcohol should be avoided and sugar, tea and coffee may hinder rather than help recovery.

Back massage and quite often massage of the hamstrings, which may also be involved, is helpful to relax the painful spasm in the back muscles. This must be done within the patient's pain tolerance which, in the early stages of an acute disc injury, may be very easily threatened.

Pulsed ultrasound for four minutes at each daily session may prove beneficial (Brearly). There are three different reactions to look for on application of ultrasound:

1. The patient experiences agonising pain within the first minute. Switch off. You may try again later and if the same response is elicited switch off and do not try again. Brearly stated that this indicates a herniated disc and the patient should be referred quickly.
2. Great reduction in pain and patient has an increase in mobility as the muscle spasm reduces. Usually the patient recovers quite quickly, although some patients tend to plateau after the first few treatments and recovery slows down.
3. Total relief of symptoms in short-term and patient goes on to full recovery after only several treatments.

My own experiences with patients has indicated that ultrasound is helpful with most patients. It helps reduce pain, inflammation and muscle spasm and once some progress is made, most patients tend to become more actively involved in their treatment and progress is good. I must also report there have been occasions when ultrasound has had neither a positive nor a negative effect upon the patient.

Resting Position

Patients usually find a position which is more comfortable for them. However, many patients find a little ease if they lie on their backs with pillows placed behind the head, perhaps under the lumbar spine, and two or even three pillows under the knees.

This position is sometimes referred to as the psoas position. It helps relaxation of the muscles of the lower abdomen and legs and eases the discomfort of many patients with disc problems.

If this is not found to be comfortable (and patients cannot be expected to remain in one position for any great length of time, anyway), I have found that a good alternative is to arrange the patient in the recovery position and place a pillow between the patient's knees. This will again, help relieve the strain.

Stretching

The patient can be encouraged to stretch even whilst bed-bound. Dr. Thomas A. Janes, a visiting lecturer to the Northern Institute, from Independence, Missouri, demonstrated a useful stretching routine for patients recovering in bed from a disc lesion.

Firstly the patient stretches out the right arm above the head as far as is comfortable. Then the left leg is stretched. Next, the patient stretches the left arm followed by the right leg.

This is exploratory and the patient is guided to perform cautiously. The next stage requires the patient to stretch the right arm and the left leg simultaneously. After a brief pause, the patient stretches the left arm and right leg at the same time.

This sequence should be repeated three times and may be performed several times each day.

Recovery from Disc Injury

Patients with severe disc injuries are comparatively rare. Usually their pain and incapacity is such that they are referred to their GP and he in turn may well refer them on to the local hospital. Here, the patient may undergo surgery.

Thus, as a general rule, the remedial therapist will not treat serious conditions until after hospital treatment. Some patients recover well after surgery; others continue to suffer and require treatment.

Many patients with less severe symptoms and conditions recover quite quickly after an initial rest of two or three days. Once the painful symptoms have eased, the patient should be encouraged to get out of bed and to begin to live as normally as possible whilst the treatment continues.

A smaller proportion of patients do not recover as quickly and it may be several weeks before they can resume even gentle activities. Some disc injuries are serious and painful and, thankfully, they are not very common. Most disc injuries respond well to the remedial treatment regime outlined in this chapter.

Hip Joint

The bones of the hip consist of three parts:

1. Pubis.
2. Ilium
3. Ischium.

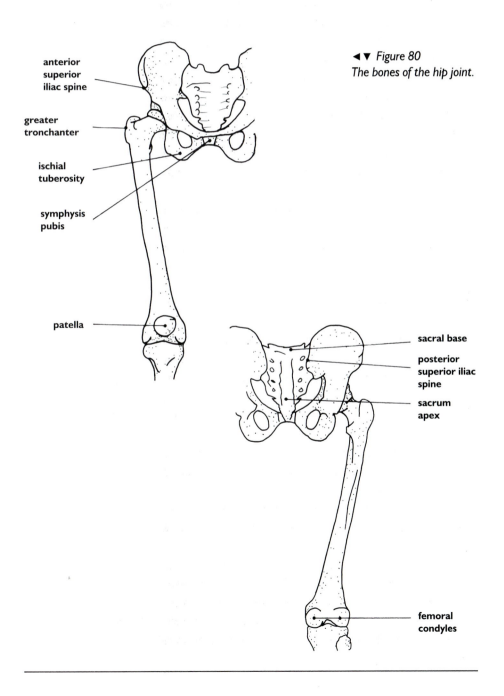

◀ ▼ *Figure 80*
The bones of the hip joint.

The bones are joined anteriorly at the symphysis pubis by a fibrous cartilage with a hyaline cartilage covering and reinforced by strong ligaments.

Posteriorly, the ilium articulates on either side with the sacrum. The sacroiliac joint is almost immovable and is reinforced by very strong ligaments.

The joint between the head of the femur and the acetabulum is a ball and socket joint. This joint has a wide range of movements; flexion, extension, abduction, adduction, medial and lateral rotation and medial and lateral circumduction.

Muscles of the Hip Joint

The anterior group includes; psoas major, iliacus which combine and become known as iliopsoas. There is a further muscle, psoas minor which is present in a substantial minority of the population. This group inserts into the region of the lesser trochanter of the femur and attaches to the last thoracic vertebra, possibly the twelfth rib, the lumbar vertebrae and their intervertebral discs, the ilium and the sacrum.

These muscles are flexors of the hip and are involved in other movements including lateral rotation and lateral bending.

The dorsal group of muscles insert into the region of the greater trochanter and include tensor fasciae latae, the gluteals maximus, medius and minimus and piriformis.

Gluteus maximus is primarily an extensor of the hip, a lateral rotator and helps prevent excessive forward tilting of the pelvis. It is also significantly involved in both abduction and adduction.

Gluteus medius is mimicked by minimus and acts in medial and lateral rotation and also in abduction in certain movements, e.g. dancing.

Piriformis originates from the pelvic surface of the sacrum and the margin of the greater sciatic notch. It passes through the greater sciatic foramen and inserts on the anteromedial aspect of the greater trochanter. It functions as a lateral rotator, an abductor and also assists in extension of the hip.

The ventral muscles function as lateral rotators and have an important function in controlling the balance of the body. They are stronger than the medial rotators and in the normal position of the limb, the apex of the foot points slightly outwards to achieve better support of the body. This group includes:

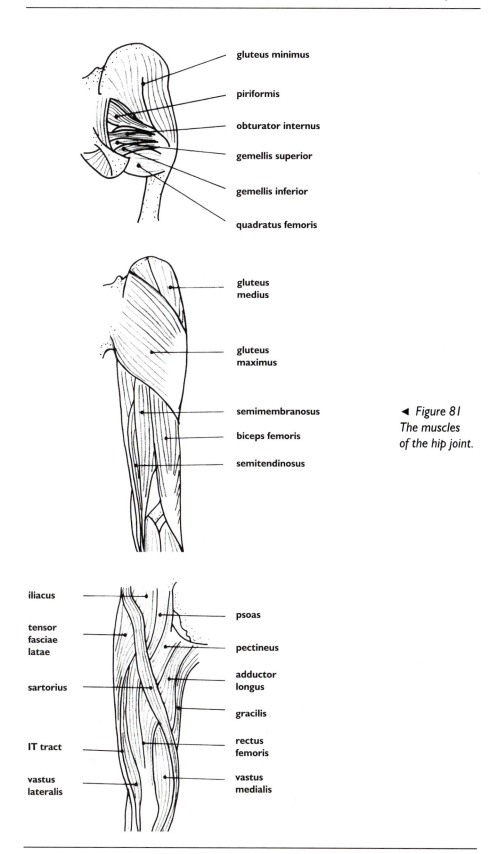

gluteus minimus

piriformis

obturator internus

gemellis superior

gemellis inferior

quadratus femoris

gluteus medius

gluteus maximus

semimembranosus

biceps femoris

semitendinosus

◀ *Figure 81*
The muscles
of the hip joint.

iliacus

tensor fasciae latae

sartorius

IT tract

vastus lateralis

psoas

pectineus

adductor longus

gracilis

rectus femoris

vastus medialis

1. Obturator internus.
2. Quadratus femoris.
3. Obturator externus.
4. Gemellus superior and inferior.

The adductor group includes:

1. Gracilis.
2. Pectineus.
3. Adductor brevis.
4. Adductor longus.
5. Adductor magnus.
6. Adductor minimus.

The adductors bring the abducted leg back to the midline and may assist in other movements including flexion (gracilis, pectineus, adductor longus), medial rotation (pectineus, adductor longus, adductor magnus, adductor minimus and extension (adductor magnus).

The posterior muscles of the hip are collectively known as the hamstrings and individually as:

1. Biceps femoris (lateral side of the leg).
2. Semitendinosus and semimembranosus (medial side of the leg).

On the anterior thigh, rectus femoris and sartorius act on both hip and knee joints. Rectus femoris assists in flexion of the hip and sartorius assists in flexion and lateral rotation of the hip.

The nerve supply to the hip is from both the lumbar and sacral plexi. The femoral nerve originates from the upper four lumbar nerves and the lumbar plexus and is distributed to the front and inner thigh.

From the sacral plexus, formed by the lower lumbar and upper sacral nerve, runs the sciatic nerve and its branches. The sciatic nerve runs posteriorly to the popliteal area where it divides into the peroneal and tibial nerves and progresses down the limb to the foot.

Hip Disorders

Children presenting with hip pain must be handled with great care. A child complaining of hip pain and unable to bear weight properly, that is, they limp may have Perthe's hip, an avascular necrosis of the femoral head. It occurs in children between the ages of four through to ten. All or part of the femoral head is affected and this patient requires expert orthopaedic treatment and should be referred, in the first instance, to the GP.

During adolescence a small percentage of children (mainly boys) may display symptoms of pain in the thigh and begin to limp. The leg may become externally rotated and show limitations in abduction and internal rotation and be shorter on comparison with the unaffected leg. The upper femoral epiphysis may have become displaced. Again, this patient must be referred to the GP prior to further treatment.

Osteoarthritis at the hip is usually associated with patients of middle age. This may not be true in some cases and younger people, especially after previous hip trauma, may develop this condition. The symptoms include:

- Pain in the groin that may radiate to the knee;
- Typically after activity at first then becoming constant;
- The discomfort may disturb sleep;
- The hip feels progressively stiffer;
- The patient develops a limp;
- The patient may feel that the affected side has a shorter leg;
- The patient develops a fixed flexion at the joint;
- Muscle wastage becomes increasingly apparent;
- Hip movements become increasingly limited;
- Greater trochanter, on affected side, appears somewhat higher and posterior;
- Painful on firm palpation.

The patient must be referred to the GP if any of these conditions are suspected by the therapist. It does not mean that the therapist is excluded from any further contribution to the treatment. However, this will very much depend upon the outcome of further examinations and, possibly, treatment.

Piriformis

The piriformis lies under gluteus maximus and functions in extension, abduction and rotation. It helps in turning and, in sport, running bends.

It lies in very close proximity to the sciatic nerve; they both pass through the same foramen. Changes in piriformis due to spasm or inflammation may result in irritation of the sciatic nerve. This may cause pain in the gluteal area and the hamstring area and may cause weakness and loss of function, for example, in walking.

Prolonged sitting may cause piriformis to spasm and affect the sciatic nerve. Examples may be found in the elderly or in workers who sit for long periods or even stand for long periods if the posture is poor. Sports people, particularly runners, are prone to piriformis problems which are often associated with overuse involving specialised activities like speed work on the track or hill repetitions.

Hip Examination

The patient may complain of pain, stiffness, the inability to walk any distance and the patient may also have developed a limp. Listen to what the patient has to say about his or her hip problem, ask questions about what the patient tells you and then delve into their medical history.

Watch the patient walk and see if it offers any clues. Better still, try to ask someone who knows the patient well if there has been a change in the patient's gait.

In a standing position, check the patient's feet for flattened arches. Changes in the structure of the feet may have significant knock-on effects not only at the hip but at other joints in the body.

Now get the patient on to the treatment table and check for any discrepancies in leg length. In the first instance, this is done by lying the patient on his back and simultaneously giving both legs a firm but gentle shaking to relax the patient. Then bring the internal malleoli together and see if they correspond or is one higher than the other. (There are more sophisticated methods of measuring leg length but the above method is a good enough first check). If there appears to be a big discrepancy the patient should be referred to a podiatrist for further examination. A discrepancy in the length of a patient's legs may be due to a number of factors:

- A congenital abnormality;
- A neurological origin;
- An infection of a bone or joint;
- A fracture of a bone, particularly if a growth zone has been affected;
- In past years, polio;
- Muscle spasm.

The first and last are perhaps the two most common ones that the therapist will encounter. A one-off leg length comparison is not always accurate. Factors taking place immediately prior to the examination may give a false first impression. My practice was next to a large supermarket and some patients combined a visit to the supermarket with a treatment. Wheeling full and uncooperative trolleys or carrying heavy shopping bags can have short-term effects on the muscles of the legs, backs and hips that may manifest in temporary leg length discrepancies.

Look for scars, swellings, wasting of muscles and the position of the limbs with the patient at rest on the table. Is one of the legs in internal rotation or is a hip slightly flexed? How do the feet settle when the patient lies down and is quite relaxed? Do the feet point at ten minutes to two on an imaginary clock or more like five minutes to three?

Palpation should be to the bony landmarks. Being able to locate the landmarks of the hip area with accuracy makes for both easier examination and treatment.

Locate the posterior iliac spine and follow it medially to the sacrum. The therapist can locate L4 vertebra in most people by placing a hand on each lateral ilium and then tracing their fingers medially to the spine. From there the therapist can palpate down to L5 vertebra and then feel the rise of the sacrum and palpate the spinous processes on the sacrum itself.

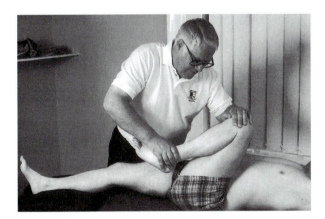

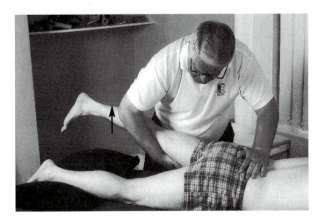

◀ *Figure 82*
(a) Passive flexion and;
(b) passive extension
of the hip.

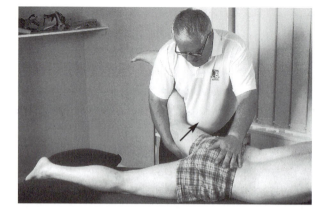

▶ *Figure 83*
Passive hip abduction.

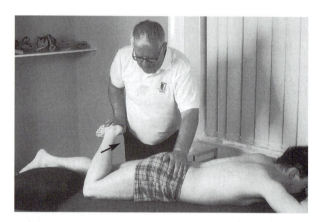

▶ *Figure 84*
(a) Passive lateral
rotation and;
(b) passive medial
rotation of the hip.

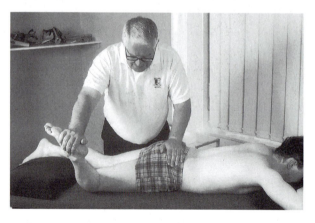

From the lateral edges of the ilia the hands can trace downwards the belly of tensor fasciae latae and then the hardness of the greater trochanter. The trochanter is hard to miss for below it the tissues become soft until the bony structures of the lateral aspect of the knee are located. The ability to locate the greater trochanter is vital to both examination and treatment.

With patient lying face down on the table, move enough of the towelling cover to expose one gluteal area. Below the curve of the gluteal group of muscles and at its junction with the posterior thigh the therapist will find, in most patients, a very definite crease between the two – the gluteal crease. Below this and at a slightly upward angle, the therapist will be able to locate the ischial tuberosity. This is the bone upon which one sits and it is also the origin of the hamstring muscles.

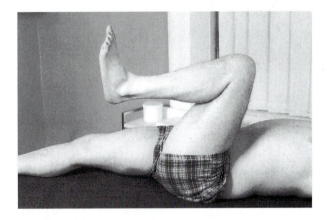

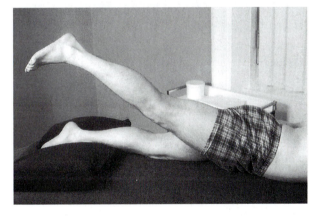

◄ *Figure 85*
(a) Active flexion and;
(b) active extension
of the hip.

These bony landmarks and muscular attachments should be palpated and the reactions of the patient noted. From this understanding, it should not be difficult to locate and palpate the bellies of the major muscles.

At this point the patient can be asked to demonstrate actively some of the movements of the hip, especially the ones that are causing trouble.

The therapist can then conduct his own examination by movement; firstly by passive movement and then by active and resisted movements. The unaffected side may also be examined by active movements to give a comparison upon which the therapist may judge the movements of the injured hip.

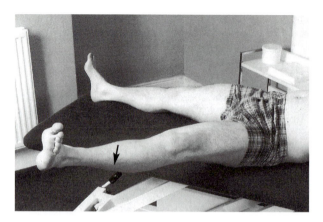

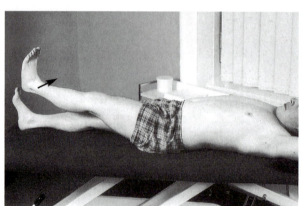

▶ *Figure 86*
(a) Active abduction and;
(b) active adduction of
the hip.

Hip Treatments

The hip does not lend itself so easily to effleurage and to obtain a relaxation of the muscles, for example, tensor fasciae latae and piriformis muscles, it may be more beneficial to employ direct pressure into the belly of the muscle. The pressure should be quite firm and held until the therapist feels the muscle relax under the weight of his fingers or thumb. This may take twenty or thirty seconds or even over a minute with some patients.

This can be followed by petrissage movements to the muscles although the effects on the deep-lying piriformis will be minimal. Piriformis can be 'goaded' by locating the belly of the muscle between its attachments and under gluteus maximus. The goading consists of deep pressure into the muscles with the fingers which are then moved back and forth across the muscle fibres.

This may also be accomplished a little more comfortably for the patient by flexing the knee with the inferior hand and taking the hip into and out of lateral and

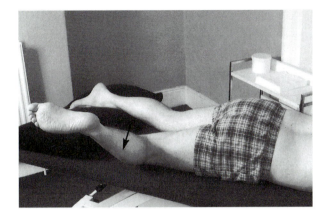

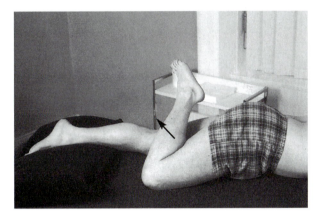

◄ Figure 87
(a) Active medial
rotation and;
(b) active lateral
rotation of the hip.

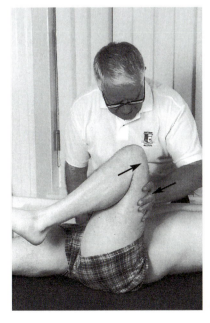

a.

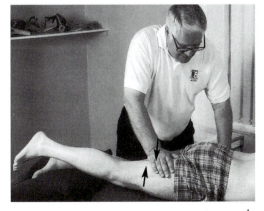

b.

◄ ▲ Figure 88
(a) Resisted flexion and;
(b) resisted extension of the hip.

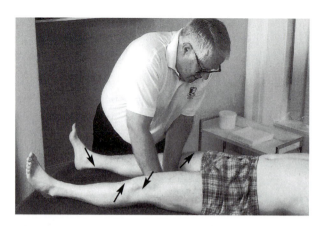

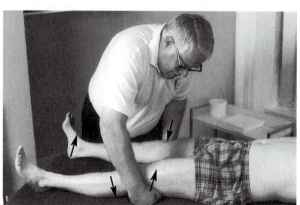

► *Figure 89*
(a) Resisted adduction
and;
(b) resisted abduction
of the hip.

medial rotation, all the while keeping the superior hand firmly pressing into the belly of piriformis.

A useful piece of advice to male patients is not to keep their wallets in the back pocket of the trousers and then to sit down for any length of time. The effects of a chunky wallet wedged into the piriformis from the hard base of a car seat has been documented many times over the years.

A technique that releases spasm from the gluteal group is known as the 'gluteal punch'. This is performed on the patient, who is lying face down on the treatment table, by the therapist who uses the middle knuckles of an 'open' fist to rhythmically and systematically punch the patient's muscles. This may take thirty or forty seconds for each side but it will depend upon individual reaction from each patient.

Most patients with hip problems will benefit by being taken through the range of passive hip movements; flexion and extension, abduction and adduction, lateral and medial rotation and circumduction. After the massage techniques have been applied, many patients show an improvement when taken through the range of passive movements.

Traction applied to the hip is beneficial, too. Traction can be applied with the patient lying face up on the table. A folded towel is placed over the anterior iliac spine to prevent discomfort to the patient.

The therapist stands at the side of the patient on which the traction is to take place. The therapist's superior hand is placed firmly on the towel that overlies the anterior superior iliac spine. The inferior arm wraps around the patient's thigh and with a steady backward pull, the traction is applied to the hip.

An easy alternative to this method, especially with an adjustable height table, is performed again with the patient lying face up on the treatment table. The therapist stands at the side of the patient awaiting traction with his legs partly flexed.

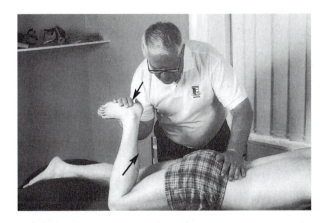

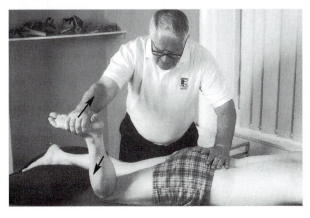

◄ *Figure 90*
(a) Resisted lateral rotation and;
(b) resisted medial rotation of the hip.

The patient is asked to flex both his hip and knee to ninety degrees. The therapist's superior hand takes a firm hold of the patient's anterior thigh just above the patella. The therapist's inferior arm is passed over the top of the patient's lower leg which it encircles and then grasps the superior arm around the wrist. Thus, the patient is firmly held by the therapist.

To help obtain maximum relaxation the patient is asked to take a deep breath and then slowly exhale. Towards the end of the exhalation, the therapist applies the traction by straightening his legs and lifting the whole of the leg upwards and tractioning the femur away from the acetabulum.

Chapter 5
Other Considerations

Arthritis

There are probably in excess of ten million people in the United Kingdom who suffer from arthritis in one of its many forms. The two most common types are osteoarthritis (O-A) and rheumatoid arthritis (R-A). There follows a brief review of some of the more common types of arthritis.

Osteoarthritis

This is the most common form of arthritis and can affect anyone, for example, Van Straten (1999) cites the example of Carl Lewis the Olympic gold medal winner, who, at the age of thirty-eight has severe arthritic problems in knees and spine. It dates back to ancient times and is found in animals as well as in humans.

It is a degenerative condition of joints in which there is a progressive destruction of the articular cartilage of the bones and the formation of new bone growth at the margins of the joint.

It is characterised by pain, stiffness, deformity and loss of function. It is usually of slow onset and many people may show signs of O-A on X-ray but not experience any of the distressing symptoms of the disease. Hands, knees and hips are commonly affected as is the spine.

Treating Patients With O-A

Many arthritic sufferers benefit from treatment by massage and movement and show improvement. The therapist should always follow a procedure of examination and assessment of each individual patient. There should be a discussion with the patient and any others already involved in the treatment of the patient regarding your future treatments.

The aims of the treatments are to ease the symptoms, to prevent further damage, to improve movement and to strengthen muscles and, importantly listed by Ward and Tidswell (1984) to maintain independence. The treatments are positive and encourage the patient to be active and positive about his or her condition.

Regular exercise is an excellent therapy to get relief from symptoms and one of the keys to joint repair listed by Campbell (1990). Activity stimulates cartilage nourishment and helps prevent further degeneration. Strong muscles offer support to joints. Avoid very heavy exercise and do not exercise joints while they are painful.

Exercise and massage are essential for the patient with ankylosing spondylitis to keep the affected joints as mobile as possible or to preserve whatever movement is left in the joints.

The various techniques of massage and heat are effective in reducing muscle spasm and easing pain. Cold treatment may be effective with some patients.

The use of passive and active movements after massage and heat are beneficial in improving movement at the joints. This may be followed by more active and then resisted movements to improve muscular strength.

Water activities are very beneficial as the warmth and bouyancy help relieve pressure on painful joints.

Rheumatoid Arthritis

R-A is not as common as O-A and is thought to affect about one and a half million people in the United Kingdom.

The causes of R-A are unclear. It is thought to be the result of an over-reaction of the immune system which reacts against the body itself rather than help to heal it. There may be several initiating factors and there are a number of interesting theories, some of which were posed by Mansfield (1990):

*   Is it an endocrine imbalance?
*   A metabolic disease?
*   Is it caused by inappropriate diet or vitamin deficiency?
*   Problems of malabsorption and bowel health?

- Pollutants and other environmental factors?
- Is stress a cause?

The most common age of onset is between thirty-five and fifty-five and three times as many women than men become a victim. Onset is usually slow but can be acute.

Any of the synovial joints can be affected though the extremities are usually the first joints involved. An important feature is symmetry for example, both hands are affected rather than just one.

There is a process of erosion and degradation of cartilage and bone. Sometimes the process is brief but usually there is a progression to joint destruction with loss of cartilage and bone leading to deformity, subluxation, secondary degenerative changes and, possibly, fibrous ankylosis. Tendon sheaths suffer in the same way as the synovial joints and may cause tendon rupture.

The condition is accompanied by inflammation, joint capsules are stretched and all peri-articular tissues come under strain. Muscle wasting, weakened tendons and ligaments and osteoporosis are common. In summary, the symptoms are severe pain, inflammation and swelling of joints, stiffness and increasing loss of function.

R-A may also progress and affect other tissues and structures including, among others, eyes, lungs, heart, the central nervous system, urinary tract and, usually as a result of drug therapy, the digestive system. Depression is associated with both the illness and the frustration of the individual's inability to cope with daily tasks and their fears for the future.

Treating Patients with R-A

The patient with rheumatoid arthritis must be handled with the utmost care and skill. The patient's condition is often one in which massage and remedial movements are temporarily contra-indicated.

The patient should not be treated by massage and exercise whilst the condition is in an active or 'flare-up' phase but rather when the patient is in a state of comparative remission.

Massage in these circumstances is helpful and beneficial. Passive movements help maintain joint function and active movements within the patient's tolerance are to be encouraged. The patient may benefit from activities in water. Many local authorities have dedicated sessions at their swimming pools for arthritics. At these sessions the general public are excluded and water temperature is raised. The activities are under the guidance and supervision of a leader qualified in exercise or, in some areas, a physiotherapist. Care is taken to ensure that the patient exercises under qualified supervision in a warm, protected environment for a suitable period of time. This is very often the most suitable form of exercise for the patient suffering from R-A.

The R-A patient suffers from a condition that is associated with muscle weakness and wasting and requires regular exercise. This should be:

*   Within the patient's pain tolerance;
*   Have easy progression but with progress the patient should be able to notice;
*   Emphasis placed on postural re-education and the abdominal muscles;
*   Exercises should not involve weights or mechanical resistance because of possible traumatisation to vulnerable joints;
*   Daily sessions of short duration;
*   Encourage and monitor activities for the patient to perform at home in their own time.

The programme for a patient with R-A requires a delicate balance of exercise and rest stated Sayce and Fraser (1988). When joints are hot, swollen and painful the patient needs to rest but their joints may be taken through their passive range of movements once or twice a day. At other times, exercise is essential to maintain function of muscles and joints. Why Exercise? To:

*   Keep joints mobile.
*   Increase muscle strength.
*   Strengthen bones and ligaments.
*   Help prevent bone deformities.
*   Maintain nourishment in the joints.
*   Maintain and increase the ability to perform daily tasks.
*   Increase a sense of wellbeing.

Ankylosing Spondylitis

This is an inflammatory condition principally affecting the spine and sacroiliac joints. Usually found in young men and thought by Ward and Tideswell to be genetic though in some cases an environmental factor may trigger the onset of the condition.

Ankylosing spondylitis involves the synovium, articular capsule and ligament attachments to the bones. There is a bridging between vertebral bodies, i.e. bone grows alongside the intervertebral discs affecting the spinal ligaments and with fusion of vertebrae and sacroiliac joints. There is erosion at the symphysis pubis and manubrio sternum, atlanto-axial suluxation and, later, stress fractures in the vertebrae. The symptoms are:

- Low back pain and stiffness;
- Loss of the lumbar lordosis;
- The head appears to be pushed forward and shoulders rounded;
- Spinal movements become impaired and chest expansion is diminished;
- Pain on palpation of bony points;
- Neurological pain.

Other complications include problems with the eyes, cardiovascular and respiratory problems and long-term renal complications. The disease may abort at any stage or it may go into remission and return years later.

Factors Affecting Healing

When making the assessment of the patient after examination there are a number of factors that should be considered by the therapist and taken into consideration when discussing with the patient his or her condition, the type, duration and frequency of treatments:

1. If the injured area or tissue has a poor blood supply the rate of healing will be slower than areas with a plentiful blood supply. An example of this is that ligaments generally take longer to heal than muscles.
2. The age of the patient is also a significant factor. Given that there are no other factors at play, a fit twenty-year old patient will recover more quickly than a fit fifty-year old, both of whom have a similar injury. For example a strain of the gastrocnemius in a twenty-year old badminton player will generally heal significantly more quickly than a similar injury in a fifty-year old player.
3. The state of the patients' general health is important. An infection can delay healing. Certain drug treatments may suppress repair, giving a slow and weak repair in muscle, tendon and ligament injuries.
4. Deficiencies in the patient's nutrition will interfere with healing, for example a deficiency of vitamin C or zinc.

Whatever the age of the patient, regular exercise is a positive beneficial factor in healing. General exercise maintains fitness and helps avoid apathy and depression. Exercise helps keep muscles toned and strong and, along with stretching, helps scar tissue formation, maintains joint mobility, muscle balance and proprioceptive reflexes. The therapist must consider these factors when making his assessment of the patient and when formulating his treatment plan:

1. The age of the patient.
2. The patient's health and levels of fitness.
3. The patient's lifestyle.
4. The type of tissue injured.

Allow for individual differences in your deliberations. Some sixty-year olds have athletic bodies and enjoy excellent health and healthy lifestyles, whereas some thirty-year olds have poor health, bodies that have already gone to seed and whose lifestyles are not conducive to good health and, for that matter, a speedy recovery after some musculoskeletal injury. The therapist should take these factors into account when assessing patients and planning the treatment for patients.

A twenty-year old club athlete with a minor hamstring strain sustained three or four days ago will require massage, perhaps some heat treatment and stretching exercises over a fifteen to twenty-one day period. All things being equal, the athlete will be able to ease back into training after that period of time.

A veteran athlete, i.e. male 0–40 and female 0–35, will have a longer recovery period and there may be complications in his or her injury from previous problems with the hamstrings. The treatments for an athlete in this age range will probably be planned over a six-week period. At the end of six weeks the therapist should go through the full examination procedure again and, depending upon the results of this, the treatments may be extended or the athlete may return to full training. I would certainly be looking to get a 'vet' to attend for regular maintenance treatments as a method of prevention of future injury.

We presume that the athletes are fit, have no other illnesses and lead a healthy lifestyle. This is not always the case and the therapist should pursue this avenue of examination rather than taking it for granted. There has been much discussion, for example, on the sports pages of the newspapers subsequent to 'Euro 2000' comparing the lifestyles of English soccer players with that of the French and Italian players. It would seem that there is a considerable difference in lifestyles that has effects on general health, fitness, susceptibility to and recovery from injury.

What about the non-athlete and the sedentary lifestyle? What about the complications of other conditions and medication? The patients who fall into these categories will usually take longer to recover from their sprains and strains and treatments should be planned on a regular basis to meet the needs of the individual patient.

Most of the patients who telephone for an appointment are motivated by pain. Often, pain is one of the last symptoms to arrive and may be one of the first symptoms to disappear after some treatment. Many patients ignore a host of minor symptoms connected with backs, necks, knees, feet, hips and elbows, sometimes for many years. However, when pain strikes, the patient reaches for the phone.

One treatment either may make things easier or relieve the pain but the patient requires more than one treatment. One of the aims of the course of massage treatment should be to address the other symptoms and to remediate the patient's situation and condition. To do this the therapist must include mobilising and stretching in the treatment plan. For some patients, strengthening exercises are necessary to strengthen weak muscles or balance the relative strength of muscles and muscle groups to help support an injured joint, for example, the muscles around a knee joint after a ligament injury.

Patients who present themselves to the therapist with a history, perhaps, of low back pain, may make their appointment for treatment during one of their occasional troublesome phases, a 'flare-up' to quote one of my patients. It may be quite simple to relieve the patient's pain as the result of one session of massage treatment. This patient should not then be dismissed, perhaps to wait for the next period of distress. The practitioner owes it to the patient to arrange for further treatments, to do the maintenance work on a regular basis that will tend to avoid future painful episodes.

Occasionally patients are reluctant to give the time or spend money on their own maintenance. Ask these patients how much they spend on car maintenance. The amount may be many hundreds of pounds per annum, even thousands. Surely their own bodies merit at least as much attention and outlay each year.

A successful practice is built upon the firm foundation of the patients who come for these important maintenance treatments at regular intervals. A successful practitioner eventually has most of his treatment appointments booked up for several weeks ahead with just a few spaces reserved each week for the completely new patients.

Treating Children

I would not normally expect to treat children by remedial massage. Healthy, young bodies do not suffer from the same types of injury as older, more mature adult bodies. Children have a natural resilience, suppleness, an ability to stretch and twist and turn, great flexibility. Most of their injuries are cuts and bruises and they heal quickly; more serious problems are usually treated by their GP or at hospital.

Colleagues at the London and Counties Society of Physiologists Education and Research Tiny Tim Centre at Coventry have a growing reputation for the treatment of children (and some adults) with handicapping conditions. Their work is currently the subject of a research programme being undertaken by the University of Coventry and we await the eventual publication of their report. The treatment of children with special needs is really outside the remit of this book.

I have found that, on occasions, parents who were already patients of mine would bring in their children for examination and possibly for treatment. I listened to an interesting illustrated lecture given by an orthopaedic consultant (Mr. J. Fairclough, FRCS of Cardiff) several years ago at the LCSP annual conference at Blackpool. One of his statements stayed in my mind; it was that, "No child should limp." If a child limps, it may be an early signal that there is something seriously amiss.

If a parent brings a child for examination, the therapist must be aware that the child may exhibit symptoms of a condition that could be potentially very serious. I refer to conditions like Osgood-Schlatter's disease, or Perthe's hip or slipped upper femoral epythysis.

Practitioners must be aware of the existence of these and other conditions, aware of the implications of these conditions for the child's future health. Examine the child by all means but the parent (who must be present at the examination) must be advised to also take the child to their family doctor for more specialised examination. The doctor will then make his diagnosis and make arrangements for the child's treatment. There must be no prevarication in these circumstances. Any child who presents to a remedial therapist with a painful hip, knee, foot, unable to bear weight properly that has been present for several days and for which there is no obvious cause must be referred to their GP.

I worked for a period of several years in a children's hospital in Manchester and I remember that one of the orthopaedic wards was kept very busily employed treating children with these conditions. The treatments often involved months, even years of skilled medical attention aimed at eventual recovery. The GP will in all probability refer your patient to a paediatric department for their expert examination, diagnosis and treatment and thank you for being aware and professional enough to refer the patient to him in the first place.

Osgood-Schlatter's disease is a reasonably common knee problem with early teenagers and Macnicol (1995) reported that of 1,000 consecutive cases of knee disorders referred to an Edinburgh clinic, some 17% were Osgood-Schlatter's disease.

I have treated, with parental and medical approval, many cases of Osgood-Schlatter's disease. Each case is different and each child requires individual treatment and management. In each case I have made certain that the child concerned has been examined at least by their own GP and that the GP's approval had been gained for my treatment.

Treatment is directed to the extensor muscles and to the attachment of the quadriceps into the lower leg at the tibial tubercle. In passing, it is perhaps worth mentioning that, when treating some elderly male patients, evidence of an incidence, many years previously, of 'Osgood's' is distinctly palpable at the tibial tubercle. The elderly men have never heard of Osgood-Schlatter's disease but are quite surprised when you ask if they had 'growing pains' when they were young lads!

The patient must rest from any activities that aggravate the condition and this sometimes causes problems, for instance, with a child's school. It may mean that an important member of the school's sports teams has an enforced absence for many months. This presents difficulties for the child, teachers, parents and peers and has to be handled in a sympathetic, collaborative manner. It may even mean that a child has to have special arrangements to prevent him climbing several flights of stairs each day at change of lessons because this brings on the pains at the knee. The period of treatment is open-ended; it may be for two or three months or much longer in some cases.

In the acute stage the aim is to reduce the pain, swelling and heat at the tibial insertion of the quadriceps. Cold application, e.g. crushed ice applied in a plastic bag for fifteen minutes at two hourly intervals. I have supplemented this with a topical application of one of the proprietary ointments or gels, for example *Enzyme Ice*, homoeopathic *Ruta Grav* or the excellent haemorrhoid ointment, *Lasonil*. Rest from activities that cause any pain is most important at this stage.

Remedial massage, i.e. effleurage and petrissage is given to both the quadriceps and hamstring group with the intention of relaxing the muscles and draining any exudate from around the knee joint. In most cases the children concerned received two or three massage sessions each week.

As the pain and swelling and inflammation are brought under control and recede, a little gentle stretching of all the muscle groups of the thigh is introduced progressively.

We now approach what are sometimes dangerous times during the treatment period. The patient is beginning to feel normal, i.e. pain free. The temptation of an impromptu game of football in the park may be difficult to resist but if the temptation is not resisted the condition returns with a vengeance. I recall the case of an unfortunate thirteen year old who followed all the advice and instructions for nearly six months. However, all his work, and mine, was undone by a group of fifteen year old bullies who threatened and then chased him for over a mile before he reached the sanctuary of his front door.

Many children recover well from Osgood-Schlatter's disease but others are handicapped to a greater or lesser degree for the rest of their lives. Some have very visible and tangible evidence. One fourteen year old boy, a footballer and athlete of some local note, was brought, hopping and clutching, into my treatment room with the worse possible set of symptoms. It looked as if the patellar ligament had become detached from the tibia. On questioning the patient and mother I discovered that the knee crisis had actually occurred almost a week previously whilst the family were away at a holiday centre. The child had received no medical attention whatsoever because, according to mum, "It didn't seem much and we were on holiday." He did, however, receive a lot of hospital treatment over the next three years and his knee did not allow him to play football again.

Treat children with great care and be prepared to refer to the child's medical practitioner if you have any doubts or worries whatsoever about that child's condition. Time may be of the greatest importance in this case.

Some of the saddest cases I have had to deal with have involved teenagers with serious knee conditions brought about by over-training, especially on hard surfaces, and over-participation in sport. Very often a boy or girl who is an excellent runner is also good at soccer or netball, may be an exceptional gymnast or trampoliner and a gifted swimmer. The pressure may be on the individual to take part in school teams and club teams and, in some cases, town or county representation. The children concerned often are involved in hard and demanding training for and participation in, two or three competitive sports simultaneously.

Many young swimmers get up at five o'clock in the morning three or four times a week to train. They may also, for instance, do athletics training two or three times each week. Muscles and joints begin to suffer in the face of unrelenting hard work and competition with insufficient recovery time. The blame is not usually with the young athlete but rather with coaches, managers, parents and teachers.

Having that child in the treatment room and examining a stressed and strained knee joint is a sombre experience for the therapist as well as the child. In some cases you instinctively know after listening to the child's history that the child will require surgical help and will not recover enough to participate at their chosen level again. Further examination by palpation and by movement serves to confirm the initial fears.

I once addressed a group of sports therapists and gave a certain patient of mine as an anonymous example of this problem. At the conclusion of the evening, several of the therapists swooped on me and all had recognised the patient. This patient had been hawked from one therapist to another by parents who refused to accept any bad news about their child's knee. As soon as the word 'rest' was mentioned they made evasive noises and withdrew their child on a quest for a therapist who would tell them to ignore the problems with the knee and carry on training. The father once said to this particular child, within earshot of a therapist, that this bit of pain in the knee was a small repayment for all the money that he spent on the child's equipment and training.

Emergency and Acute Conditions

It is unwise to think that emergency situations arise only in the sphere of sports injury work and that the therapist who works from his or her own treatment room or clinic is at a safe distance from the 'emergency patient'. The newly qualified therapist will soon encounter situations in which a patient requires urgent, expert medical treatment and a skilled professional to make the necessary arrangements and look after the patient until that help arrives. This may happen in the clinic, by chance in a public place or at a function.

During my own clinical days I was called upon to deal with patients suffering heart attacks, patients with fractured limbs and, on one occasion, spinal fractures. Also, patients in diabetic comas and with epileptic fits; road accident victims on the main road outside; a child bitten by a dog in the street; a scaffolder on a nearby roof with a back spasm; a drunk with a head injury and countless passers-by with all manner of injury who found my clinic to be convenient.

All therapists should have a current First Aid qualification. Patients may present to you with symptoms that demand that you get urgent medical help for them:

- Persistent headaches, nausea, dizziness, vomiting, lapsing into unconsciousness after a head injury.
- Breathing difficulties, especially after a blow to the head, neck or chest.
- Pains in the neck after an impact.
- Abdominal pains after an injury situation.
- Blood in the urine and especially after an injury situation.
- Obvious or suspected fracture.
- Severe or suspected severe ligament injury.
- Joint dislocation.
- Eye injury.
- Deep wound.

- Wound which shows no sign of stopping bleeding.
- Intense, unremitting pain.
- Injury about which there are doubts regarding the severity and diagnosis.
- Persisting and severe symptoms from a muscle or joint injury.

Head Injury

A patient may present to you with a history of very recent head injury, for example, sustained during a sporting event or as the result of a fall at home. In some cases of head injury, the symptoms are not apparent for up to twenty-four hours. You may need to refer the patient to hospital or their own GP if any of the following are present:

- Dizziness and/or loss of co-ordination after injury.
- Temporary loss of memory and or confusion after the injury.
- Severe, deep throbbing headache.
- Blurred or double vision.
- Ringing noises in ears.
- Unequal pupil sizes.
- No pupil reaction to light.
- Slurred speech.
- Convulsions or tremor.
- Nausea or vomiting.
- Sleepiness or 'grogginess'.
- Difficulty in being woken.
- Fluid seeping from nose and/or ears.
- Partial or complete paralysis or numbness.

Summary

In an emergency situation the therapist's function is to re-assure the patient, to offer comfort, to make sure that the patient is not in any further dangers, to keep the patient warm and, most importantly, to summon expert help.

Glossary of Terms

Abduction

Lateral movement away from the midline of the body.

Acute

In remedial massage, this term is used for the early stages of an injury.

Adduction

Medial movement towards the midline of the body.

Agonist

A muscle or muscles responsible for joint movement, also known as prime mover.

Amphiarthrosis

A joint with slight movement that connects bone to bone with a fibrocartilage or hyaline cartilage.

Anatomy

The study of the structures of the body.

Antagonist

The opposite of agonist (above). A muscle or group of muscles having the opposite action to the prime mover or agonist but which work with the agonist by relaxing muscle(s) and allowing movement to take place.

Aorta

The artery that carries blood out of the heart.

Arteriole

The smallest type of artery.

Artery

Blood vessels that carry oxygenated blood from the heart to the body.

Arthritis

The commonest type of joint disorder and usually refers to wear and tear of a joint. There are many varieties, e.g. osteo- and rheumatoid arthritis, perhaps the two most commonly known.

Articulation

Another word for a joint.

Atrophy

A decrease in the size of a tissue or organ, often caused in musculoskeletal structures by lack of use.

Attachments

Referred to also as the origins and insertions of muscles; where skeletal muscles are connected to bones.

Avulsion

The tearing away of one part from another, e.g. ligament from bone.

Axilla

An armpit.

Ball and Socket Joint

A ball-shaped convex surface fitted into a concave socket.

Bursa

A small sac of fibrous tissue containing synovial fluid situated where parts move upon one another at a joint to reduce friction.

Capillary

A minute blood vessel.

Cardiac Muscle

Striated involuntary muscle fibres in the heart.

Carpus

The eight bones of the wrist.

Cartilage

Fibrous connective tissue, e.g. hyaline cartilage, elastic cartilage and fibrocartilage.

Central Nervous System

The brain and the spinal cord.

Cerebrospinal Fluid

A clear colourless fluid that flows throughout the brain and around the spinal cord.

Chronic   Of long duration.

Chronic Pain   Pain that continues over a long
                                     period of time.

Circumduction   Circular movement at a joint combining
                                     the movements of flexion, extension,
                                     abduction, adduction and rotation.

Compact Bone   The hard portion of bone.

Concentric Contraction   The action of a prime mover where a muscle
                                     develops tension as it shortens in order to
                                     provide enough force to overcome resistance.

Condyle   A rounded projection at the end of a bone.

Condyloid Joint   A joint that allows movement in
                                     two directions but one of which is
                                     usually dominant.

Connective Tissue   The tissue that holds and supports
                                     the body and its parts.

Contusion   A bruise.

Coronary Arteries   The arteries that supply oxygenated
                                     blood to the heart.

Cramp   A painful muscle spasm.

Cranial Nerves   Twelve pairs of nerves originating from the
                                     brain that transmit information to and from
                                     the sense organs of the face, facial muscles,
                                     and muscles of the neck and upper shoulders.

Dermatitis   A general term for acute or chronic
                                     skin inflammation.

Dermatone   A section of skin supplied by
                                     a single spinal nerve.

Dermis   The inner layer of the skin.

Diagnosis   Determination of the nature of a disease
                          or condition by the study of the signs
                          and symptoms.

Diaphragm   A dome-shaped sheet of muscle attached
                          to the thoracic wall that separates the
                          lungs from the abdominal cavity.

Diarthrosis   A freely movable synovial joint.

Disease   A definite pathological process having a
                          characteristic set of signs and symptoms.

Dorsiflexion   Movement of the ankle that results in the
                          foot moving towards the anterior tibia.

Efferent Nerves   Nerves that link the central nervous system
                          to the effectors outside the central nervous
                          system and transmit motor impulses.

Elevation   Upward movement.

Endocrine Gland   A ductless gland that secretes hormones
                          directly into the bloodstream.

Epicondyle   A projection of bone above a condyle.

Epithelial Tissue   Specialised tissue that covers and protects
                          and usually found in areas where substances
                          move into and out of the body during
                          secretion, absorption and excretion.

Eversion   The movement of the sole of the foot
                          away from the midline.

Exocrine Gland   A gland that secretes hormones directly
                          through ducts to specific parts of the body.

Extension   A movement that increases the angle
                          between two bones.

Fibrocartilage	A connective tissue that permits little motion in joints and structures.
Fibromyalgia	A condition that has symptoms of widespread pain, fatigue, poor sleep, and morning stiffness.
Fibrous Joint	A joint at which fibrous tissue connects bone directly to bone.
Flaccid	Describes a muscle lacking tone.
Flexion	A movement that decreases the angle between two bones.
Foramen	An opening in a bone.
Fossa	A depression in a bone.
Gait	The movement of the legs, trunk and arms in walking.
Ganglion	A round cyst usually not painful located on tendon sheaths or joint capsules.
Gliding Joint	A joint that only allows a gliding movement.
Haemoglobin	The oxygen carrying protein molecule within the red blood cells.
Heart	The pump of the cardiovascular system.
Heart Rate	The number of cardiac cycles in one minute, usually between 60 and 70 per minute in a healthy adult.
Hernia	A protusion of any part of the internal organs through the structures enclosing them.
Hinge Joint	Allows the movements of flexion and extension in one direction.

Hyaline Cartilage

The covering of articular connective tissue on the ends of bones in freely moveable joints in the adult skeleton.

Hyperextension

A movement that takes a part further than usual in the direction of extension.

Hypermobility

The range of movement of a joint is more than normally found in the structure.

Hypomobility

The range of movement of a joint is less than normally found in the structure.

Inflammation

The protective response of the tissues to injury or irritation that may be acute or chronic.

Insertion

The distal attachment of a muscle.

Inversion

The movement of the sole of the foot inward towards the midline.

Ischaemia

A deficiency of blood supply to a part of the body.

Isometric Contraction

The action of the prime mover that occurs when tension develops within the muscle but no appreciable change occurs in the joint angle or length of the muscle. Movement does not occur.

Isotonic Contraction

The action of the prime mover that occurs when tension is developed in the muscle while it either shortens or lengthens.

Joint Capsule

The structure of connective tissue that connects the bony components of a joint.

Kyphosis

Posterior curvature of the spine and often used to denote an excessive curvature of the thoracic spine.

Ligament

Connective tissue, mainly collagen, that connects bones and strengthens and stabilises joints.

Lordosis

The curve of the lumbar spine and often used to describe an excessive forward curve of the lumbar spine.

Lymph

A clear interstitial fluid that bathes the cells; part of the immune response; returns plasma proteins that have leaked out through capillary walls; transports fats from the gastrointestinal system to the bloodstream.

Matrix

The basic substance between the cells of a tissue.

Melanin

The pigment that colours our skin and works as a natural sunscreen to protect us from UV rays.

Membrane

A thin elastic tissue covering the surface of certain organs and lining the cavities of the body.

Metabolism

The physical and chemical processes in the body that convert food and oxygen into energy to support growth, distribute nutrients and eliminate waste products.

Mixed Nerves

A nerve that contains both sensory and motor axons.

Mole

A benign pigmented skin growth.

Motor Point

The place where the motor neuron enters the muscle, usually in the muscle belly.

Neoplasm

A tumour (may be benign or malignant).

Nerve

A bundle of conducting fibres enclosed in a sheath called the epineurium.

Nociceptors

Sensory receptors that detect painful or intense stimuli.

Opposition

The movement made by the thumb to make contact with the fingers.

Origin

The least movable attachment of a muscle; the proximal attachment.

Pain

A feeling of distress, suffering or agony caused by stimulation of specialised nerve endings.

Pathology

The study of disease, especially of the structural and functional changes in tissue and organs which cause or are caused by disease.

Pericardium

The double membranous serous sac surrounding the heart.

Periosteum

The thin membrane of connective tissue that covers bones except at articulations.

Peripheral Nervous System

Comprises the afferent (sensory) division and the efferent (motor) division.

Phantom Pain

Pain or other sensation experienced in a missing part after limb amputation.

Physiology

The study of the functions and processes of the living body.

Pivot Joint

A joint that allows rotation around the length of a bone.

Plantar Flexion

The movement of the ankle that results in the foot moving away from the body.

Plasma

A straw coloured fluid that constitutes 55% of the blood.

Plexus

A network of nerves that innervates a region of the body.

Process

A prominent projection from a bone.

Pronation

Turning the palm of the hand downwards.

Prone

Lying face down.

Proprioceptors

Sensory nerves that supply the body with information about position, movement, joint activity, muscle tension and equilibrium.

Psoriasis

A chronic disease of the skin that is characterised by redness and dry scales.

Pulmonary Vein

A vein that brings oxygenated blood from the lungs to the heart.

Referred Pain

Pain felt at some distance from its original site.

Reflex

An automatic reaction to a stimulus.

Respiration

The breathing process.

Rotation

A movement of partial turning by pivoting in an arc around a central axis.

Rupture

Tearing of connective tissue fibres.

Saddle Joint

A joint that is convex in one plane and concave in the other.

Sesamoid Bone

Round bones that are found embedded in tendons and joint capsules.

Spinal Cord

The portion of the CNS that emerges from the skull into the spinal canal.

Spinal Nerve

There are 31 pairs of mixed nerves that originate in the spinal cord and emerge from the vertebral column.

Stress

Any factor, mental or physical, the pressure of which can adversely affect the functioning of the body.

Sub-acute

A stage between acute and chronic applied to the characteristics of a disease or condition.

Supine

Lying with the face up.

Sympathetic Nervous System

That part of the autonomic nervous system that provides for most of the body's active functions.

Symphysis

A cartilaginous joint in which the bones are joined by a plate or disc of fibrocartilage.

Synarthrosis

A non-synovial joint.

Synergist

A muscle that aids or assists the action of the prime mover but is not principally responsible for the movement.

Synovial Fluid

A thick, colourless fluid secreted by the membranes of the joint cavity.

Synovial Joint

A freely moving joint that has movement in one or more planes of action.

Tendinitis

Inflammation of a tendon.

Tenosynovitis

Inflammation of a tendon sheath.

Thorax

The chest cavity.

Tone

A state of slight contraction found in skeletal muscles that enables the muscle to respond to stimulation.

Trochanter   Bony processes found on the femur.

Tubercle   A small rounded process of bone.

Tuberosity   A large rounded protuberance on a bone.

Ulcer   A round open sore of the skin or
                                    mucous membrane.

Veins   Blood vessels that primarily return blood
                                    from the capillaries and return it to the heart.

Whiplash Injury   An injury to the neck which results
                                    from a sudden thrusting forwards and
                                    snapping back of the unsupported head.

Bibliography and References

American Journal of Epidemiology: 1975.

Andry, M.: in Keith, A., 1919.

Apley, A. G., and Solomon, L.: 1997. Physical Examinations in Orthopaedics. Butterworth-Heinemann, Oxford.

Benjamin, P. J., and Lamp, S. P.: 1996. Understanding Sports Massage. Human Kinetics, Champaign, Il.

Bernieri, F.: 2000. Daily Mail, 15.6.00

BMA: 1993. Medical Ethics Today. The British Medical Association, London.

Brearley, I.: 1988. Ultrasound Techniques. Brearley, Burton-on-Trent.

Briggs, J.: 2000. Sports Therapy Diploma Course. Northern Institute of Massage.

Cailliet, R.: 1991. Shoulder Pain. F. A Davis, Philadelphia.

Cailliet, R.: 1992. Knee Pain and Disability. F. A Davis, Philadelphia.

Campbell, G. W.: 1990. A Doctor's Proven Home Cure for Arthritis. Guild Publishing, London.

Carter: 2000

Cassar, M-P.: 1999. Handbook of Massage Therapy. Butterworth-Heinemann, Oxford.

Despard, L. L.: 1916. Textbook of Massage and Remedial Gymnastics, 2nd ed. Oxford Medical, Oxford.

Duncombe, S.: 1970. Neuromuscular Massage: Supplementary Seminar Notes. Northern Institute of Massage.

Edeling, J.: 1988. Manual Therapy for Chronic Headache. Butterworth-Heinemann, Oxford.

Evans, P.: 1988. The Knee Joint. Churchill Livingstone, Edinburgh.

Field, D.: 1997. Anatomy: Palpation and Surface Markings. Butterworth-Heinemann, Oxford.

Field, T.: 2000. Touch Therapy. Churchill Livingstone, Edinburgh.

Goldstone, L.: 1999. From Orthodox to Complementary: the Fall and Rise of Massage, With Specific Reference to Orthopaedic and Rheumatology Nursing. *Journal of Orthopaedic Nursing*, 3, 152-159.

Goldstone, L.: 2000. Massage as an Orthodox Medical Treatment: Past and Future. *Complementary Therapies in Nursing and Midwifery*. November, 2000.

Goodall-Copestake, B. M.: 1917. The Theory and Practice of Massage. H. K. Lewis and Co., London.

Graham, D.: 1884. Practical Treatise on Massage. Wm. Wood, New York.

Greenman, P. E.: 1989. Principles of Manual Medicine. Williams and Wilkins, Baltimore.

Halliday, G.: 2000. Deep Lymphatic Therapy: Course Notes. Northern Institute of Massage.

Harper, B. B.: 1999. Back to Basics: Course Notes. Northern Institute of Massage.

Health and Safety Executive. 2001.

Hodkinson, 2000. Blue Moon. Mainstream Sport.

Hoppenfield, S.: 1976. Physical Examinations of the Spine and Extremities. Appleton Century Crofts, Norwalk, Connecticut.

Hungerford, M.: 1991. Beyond Sports Medicine. Sports Massage Training Institute. Costa Mesa CA.

Hungerford, M.: 1998. Sports Massage: Course Notes. Northern Institute of Massage.

Jackson, A. J.: 1993. Massage Therapy. Optima, London.

Janes, T. A.: 1994. Thirty Years in a Volume Practice. Janes, Independence, Mo.

Keith, A.: 1919. Menders of the Maimed. Hodder & Stoughton, London.

King, R. K.: 1993. Performance Massage. Human Kinetics, Champaign, Il.

Lachman, S.: 1988. Soft Tissue Injuries in Sport. Blackwell, Oxford.

McDonald, G.: 1999. Medicine Hands. Findhorn Press, Forres.

McIlwraith, B.: 1993. An Analysis of the Driving Position in the Modern Motor Car. *British Osteopathic Journal*. Vol XI, 27–34.

Macnicol, M. F.: 1998. The Problem Knee. Butterworth-Heinemann, Oxford.

Mansfield, J.: 1990. Arthritis: the Allergy Connection. Thorsons, Wellingborough.

Meager, J.: 1990. Sports Massage. Station Hill Press, New York.

Menon, P. and Asokananda, D.: 1999. One Rope, Two Feet and Healing Oils. D. K. Editions, Duang Kamol.

Mitchell, A. and Cormack, M.: 1998. The Therapeutic Relationship in Complementary Health Care. Churchill Livingstone, Edinburgh.

Dix, H., Knuttgen, H.G., Tittel, K.: 1988. The Olympic Book of Sports Medicine. Blackwell, Oxford.

Porter, R.: 1997. The Greatest Benefit to Mankind. Harper Collins, London.

Reilly, 1998.

Rosser, M.: 1996. Body Massage. Hodder and Stoughton, London.

Salvo, S. G.: 1999. Massage Therapy. W. B. Saunders, Philadelphia.

Sanderson, M.: 2000. Soft Tissue Release - a Practical Handbook for Physical Therapists. Corpus Publishing Limited, Chichester.

Sayce, V., Fraser, I.: 1988. Exercise Beats Arthritis. Thorsons, Wellingborough.

Seager, A.: 2000. Two Feet From Our Thoughts. LTS Publishing, Bristol.

Tappan, F. M.: 1988. Healing Massage Techniques. Appleton and Lange, Norwalk, Connecticut.

Tod, E. M.: 1951. Massage and Medical Gymnastics. Churchill, London.

Tucker, W. E.: 1969. Home Treatment and Posture. E & S Livingstone, Edinburgh.

Van Straten, M.: 1999. Daily Express, "Lewis the Track Hero With an Old Man's Joints." 10.6.99.

Walker, A.: 1995. Patient Compliance and the Placebo Effect. *Physiotherapy*, March, 81:3.

Ward, D. J., Tidwel,l M. E.: 1984. In Cash's Textbook of Orthopaedics and Rheumatology for Physiotherapists. Faber and Faber, London.

Wiener, S. L.: 1993. Differential Diagnosis of Acute Pain. McGraw-Hill, New York.

Woodward, K.: 1967. The Art of Massage. Northern Institute of Massage.

Useful Addresses

Training Organisations, Accredited Tutors and Professional Bodies

Northern Institute of Massage
14–16 St. Mary's Place
Bury
BL9 0DZ
Tel/fax: 0161 797 1800
www.nim56.co.uk

Kieran Corcoran
Northern Institute of Massage Tuition Centre
Cedars Osteopathic Clinic
Falvey's Health Studio
Nicholas Well Lane
Blarney Street
CORK

Michael Kerr
Northern Institute of Massage Tuition Centre
Bodycare Injury Clinic
10 Hatmore Park
LONDONDERRY
BT48 0AZ

Kirsty Muir and Nicola Pittman
Northern Institute of Massage Tuition Centre
16 Coul Park
ALNESS, Ross-shire
IV17 0XB

Franz Browne
Holistic Centre
Farms Estate
Charlestown
Nevis
West Indies

Joyce Raiwet
Box 38
Clyde
Alberta
Canada
TOG 0PO

Alexander Adamidis
89 Keas Street
Athens 11255
Greece

Michael Changkye
19 Brodie Street
Beau-Bassin
MAURITIUS

Professional Body for Massage and Manipulative Therapists

The London and Counties Society of Physiologists (LCSP)
330 Lytham Road
BLACKPOOL
FY4 1DW
Tel: 01253 408443

The LCSP Education and Research Development (ERD) Tiny Tim Centre
Whitefriars Lane
COVENTRY
CV1 2DT
Tel: 02476 228254

SUPPLIERS

Alexandra Workwear

3 Hanover Square
London
W15 1HD
Tel: 020 7 723 9906

Bretherton Therapy Products

29 Orchard Road
Beeston
Sandy
SG19 1PJ
Tel: 01767 680041

Darley Couches

5 Restormel Estate
Lostwithiel
PL22 OHG
Tel: 01208 873200

Duffield Medical

4–6 Knowsley Road
Haslingden
BB4 4RX
Tel: 01706 210297

Houghton's Books

St. Mary's Old School
Gundry Lane
Bridport
DT6 3RL
Tel: 01308 420494

Portable Massage Couches

Mr. G. Kay
119 Thatch Leach Lane
Whitefield
Manchester
M45 6FN
Tel: 0161 796 5092

Russell Medical
PO Box 3
Hanley Castle
WR8 0DJ
Tel: 01684 311 444
Fax: 01684 311 555
e-mail: thetallguy@russellmedical.co.uk

Sportscare/Medisport
100 Shaw Road
Oldham
OL1 4AY
Tel: 0161 633 533

Appendix

Origins, Insertions and Actions of Muscles

Some Muscles Acting on the Hand and Forearm

MUSCLE	ORIGIN	INSERTION	ACTION
abductor digiti minimi	pisiform and tendon of flexor carpi ulnaris	proximal phalanx of little finger	abducts little finger
abductor pollicis brevis	tubercle of scaphoid, tubercle of trapezium, flexor retinaculum	proximal phalanx of thumb	abducts and flexes thumb
abductor pollicis longus	ulna, radius and interosseous membrane	base of 1st metacarpal	abducts and extends thumb
adductor pollicis 1. oblique head 2. transverse head	2nd and 3rd metacarpals, capitate, trapezoid 3rd metacarpal	base of proximal phalanx of thumb	adducts and opposes thumb
anconeus	lateral epicondyle of humerus	olecranon process of ulna	extends elbow joint
biceps brachii 1. short head 2. long head	coracoid process of scapula supraglenoid tubercle of scapula	radius and deep fascia of forearm	flexes and supinates forearm
brachialis	anterior aspect of humerus	coronoid process and tuberosity of ulna	flexes elbow joint
brachioradialis	lateral supracondylar ridge of humerus	lower part of radius	flexes elbow joint
extensor carpi radialis brevis	lateral epicondyle of humerus	base of 3rd metacarpal	extends wrist
extensor carpi radialis longus	lateral supracondylar ridge of humerus	base of 2nd metacarpal	extends wrist
extensor carpi ulnaris	lateral epicondyle of humerus	base of 5th metacarpal	extends wrist
extensor digiti minimi	lateral epicondyle of humerus	proximal phalange of little finger	extends proximal joint of little finger
extensor digitorum communis	lateral epicondyle of humerus	common extensor tendon of each finger	extends wrist and proximal joints of fingers
extensor pollicis brevis	radius and interosseous membrane	base of proximal phalanx of thumb	extends proximal joint of thumb, abducts hand
extensor pollicis longus	ulna and interosseous membrane	base of distal phalanx of thumb	extends and abducts thumb
flexor carpi radialis	medial epicondyle of humerus	base of 2nd and 3rd metacarpals	flexes wrist joint

Some Muscles Acting on the Hand and Forearm

MUSCLE	ORIGIN	INSERTION	ACTION
flexor carpi ulnaris	medial epicondyle of humerus and ulna	pisiform, hamate and proximal end of 5th metacarpal	flexes wrist joint
flexor digiti minimi brevis	anterior surface of flexor retinaculum, hook of hamate	proximal phalanx of little finger	flexes proximal joint of little finger
flexor digitorum profundus	medial and anterior aspects of ulna and interosseous membrane	four tendons to distal phalanges of each finger	flexes fingers at distal joints and helps to flex wrist
flexor digitorum superficialis	medial epicondyle of humerus, coronoid process of ulna and radius	four tendons to middle phalanges of each finger	flexes middle phalanges of fingers and helps to flex wrist
flexor pollicis brevis	greater multangular and carpal ligament	proximal phalange of thumb	flexes proximal joint of thumb
flexor pollicis longus	radius and interosseous membrane, epicondyle of humerus, coronoid process of ulna	distal phalange of thumb	flexes thumb
lumbricales	tendons of flexor digitorum profundus in palm	one to each extensor tendon of fingers	flexes proximal joints and extends medial joints of fingers
palmaris brevis	flexor retinaculum and palmar aponeurosis	skin on medial side of hand	depresses hollow of hand
palmaris longus	medial epicondyle of humerus	flexor retinaculum and palmar aponeurosis	flexes hand
pronator quadratus	distal surface of ulna	distal surface of radius	pronates forearm and hand
pronator teres	medial epicondyle of humerus and coronoid process of ulna	lateral surface of radius	pronates forearm
supinator	lateral epicondyle of humerus, shaft of ulna, fascia at elbow	dorsal and lateral surface of radius	supinates forearm
triceps brachii 1. long head 2. medial head 3. lateral head	infraglenoid tuberosity shaft of humerus shaft of humerus	olecranon process of ulna	extends elbow, long head helps to adduct humerus if arm is abducted

Some Muscles of the Lower Leg and Foot

MUSCLE	ORIGIN	INSERTION	ACTION
abductor digiti minimi	calcaneum and plantar aponeurosis	proximal phalanx of little toe	abducts little toe
abductor hallucis	calcaneum, flexor retinaculum and plantar aponeurosis	medial surface of first phalanx of great toe	abducts and flexes great toe
adductor hallucis 1. oblique head 2. transverse head	2nd, 3rd and 4th metatarsals 3rd, 4th and 5th toes	lateral side of base of proximal phalanx of great toe	adducts great toe
extensor digitorum brevis	calcaneum	tendons of four inner toes	extends the four toes
extensor digitorum longus	head of fibula, lateral condyle of tibia	tendons of four inner toes	extends toes, dorsiflexes foot at ankle, everts foot
extensor hallucis longus	medial surface of fibula	distal phalanx of great toe	extends great toe and inverts foot
flexor digitorum brevis	calcaneum	sides of middle phalanx of 2nd-5th toes	flexes toes
flexor digitorum longus	tibia	base of distal phalanx of 2nd-5th toes	flexes toes, inverts foot
flexor hallucis brevis	cuboid, lateral cuneiform bone	proximal phalanx of great toe	flexes great toe
flexor hallucis longus	shaft of fibula	distal phalanx of great toe	flexes great toe, inverts foot
gastrocnemius	femur	calcaneum by Achilles tendon	plantar flexes foot and flexes knee joint
interossei, dorsal	metatarsal bones	extensor tendons of four toes	abducts toes
interossei, plantar	metatarsal bones	extensor tendons of 3rd-5th toes	adducts toes
peroneus brevis	lateral surface of fibula	5th metatarsal	everts and plantar flexes foot
peroneus longus	lateral surface of fibula	1st metatarsal and cuneiform	supports arches. Everts and plantar flexes foot
peroneus tertius	anterior surface of fibula	5th metatarsal	everts and dorsiflexes foot
plantaris	femur	calcaneum, by Achilles tendon	plantar flexes foot and flexes leg
soleus	fibula and tibia	calcaneum, by Achilles tendon	plantar flexes foot
tibialis anterior	upper part of tibia	1st metatarsal and cuneiform	dorsiflexes and inverts foot
tibialis posterior	tibia and fibula	tuberosity of navicular, cuboid, cuneiforms and 2nd-4th metatarsals	plantar flexes and inverts foot. Supports arches.

Some Muscles Acting on the Knee Joint

MUSCLE	ORIGIN	INSERTION	ACTION
biceps femoris	femur and ischial tuberosity	fibula head, lateral condyle of tibia	flexes knee joint; extends hip joint (by head of muscle)
gastrocnemius	femur	calcaneum, by Achilles tendon	plantar flexes ankle and flexes knee joint
gracilis	pubis	tibia (medial surface)	adducts femur, flexes knee
plantaris	femur	calcaneum, by Achilles tendon	plantar flexes foot, flexes leg
popliteus	femur (lateral condyle)	tibia	flexes knee and medially rotates leg
rectus femoris	ilium	patella and tibia	extends knee joint and flexes hip
sartorius	ilium	tibia	flexes hip and knee; laterally rotates femur
semimembranosus	ischial tuberosity	tibia (medial condyle)	flexes knee and extends hip
semitendinosus	ischial tuberosity	tibia (medial aspect)	flexes knee and extends hip
tensor fasciae latae	outer iliac crest	iliotibial tract	abducts and rotates thigh, draws fascia lata up which stabilises the knee
vastus intermedius	femur	patella and tibia	extends knee
vastus lateralis	greater trochanter	patella	extends knee
vastus medialis	femur	patella and tibia	extends knee

Muscles of the Hip

MUSCLE	ORIGIN	INSERTION	ACTION
adductors (longus, brevis, magnus)	pubis and ischium	linea aspera and supracondylar line	adducts, extends, flexes femur
biceps femoris	ischial tuberosity and linea aspera	head of fibula and lateral condyle of tibia	extends hip and flexes knee
gemelli	spine and ischial tuberosity	tendon of obturator internus	rotates femur laterally
gluteus maximus	posterior gluteal line of ilium and crest above and also sacrum and coccyx	fascia lata and gluteal tuberosity of femur	abducts, extends and laterally rotates hip, extends trunk
gluteus medius	between posterior and middle gluteal lines of ilium	greater trochanter	abducts femur and rotates thigh medially
gluteus minimus	between middle and inferior gluteal lines of ilium	greater trochanter	abducts femur and rotates thigh medially
iliopsoas	12th thoracic and all lumbar vertebrae, iliac fossa and front of sacrum	lesser trochanter	flexes hip and rotates femur medially
obturator externus	outer pubis, ischium and obturator membrane	trochanteric fossa of femur	rotates femur laterally
obturator internus	inner surface of pelvis	greater trochanter	rotates femur laterally
piriformis	front of sacrum	greater trochanter	rotates femur laterally, abducts thigh
quadratus femoris	ischium	intertrochanteric crest	rotates femur laterally
quadriceps femoris	iliac spine, acetabulum, greater trochanter, linea aspera, intertrochanteric line, gluteal tuberosity, suprocondylar line	tibial tuberosity, patella	extends knee and flexes hip joint
semimembranosus	ischium	medial condyle of tibia	extends hip and flexes knee
tensor fasciae latae	outer iliac crest	iliotibial tract	abducts and rotates thigh

Muscles of the Shoulder

MUSCLE	ORIGIN	INSERTION	ACTION
infraspinatus	infraspinous fossa of scapula	greater tuberosity	laterally rotates and abducts arm
latissimus dorsi	lower 6 thoracic vertebrae and through lumbo-dorsal fascia from lumbar vertebrae and iliac crest	bicipital groove of humerus	extends, adducts and medially rotates arm, draws shoulder downward and backward
levator scapulae	upper 4 cervical vertebrae	upper part of vertebral border of scapula	elevates shoulder and rotates scapula
rhomboideus major	2-5th thoracic vertebrae	medial border of scapula	retracts and stabilises scapula, assists in adduction of the arm
rhomboideus minor	ligamentum nuchae and 1st thoracic vertebra	medial border of scapula	retracts and stablises scapula, rotates scapula (assists in adduction of the arm)
serratus anterior	upper 8 or 9 ribs	costal surface of medial border of scapula	draws shoulder forward and rotates scapula
subclavius	1st rib	clavicle	draws shoulder downward and forward
subscapularis	subscapular fossa of scapula	lesser tuberosity of humerus	medially rotates arm
supraspinatus	supraspinous fossa of scapula	greater tuberosity of humerus	abducts arm and helps steady the head of humerus
teres major	inferior angle of scapula	medial lip of bicipital groove of humerus	medially rotates, adducts and extends arm
teres minor	axillary border of scapula	greater tuberosity of humerus	laterally rotates arm
trapezius	occiput, ligamentum nuchae and all thoracic vertebrae	clavicle and spine of scapula	elevates and braces shoulder and rotates scapula

Muscles of the Spine

MUSCLE	ORIGIN	INSERTION	ACTION
multifidis	ilium, sacrum and transverse process of vertebrae	spinous processes of vertebrae	extends and rotates trunk
quadratus lumborum	iliac crest and iliolumbar ligament	12th rib and transverse processes of upper 4 lumbar vertebrae	laterally flexes trunk
rotatores	transverse processes of thoracic vertebrae	base of spinous process of next vertebra above	extends and rotates trunk
sacrospinalis	sacrum and iliac crest	ribs, vertebrae and mastoid process	extends trunk - (action of one side only, flexes trunk laterally)
semispinalis capitis	lower 4 cervical and upper 6-7 thoracic vertebrae	occiput	extends and rotates neck
semispinalis cervicis and thoracis	transverse processes of thoracic vertebrae	spinous processes of vertebrae 6 or 7 above	extends and rotates trunk
splenius	lower half of ligamentum nuchae and 1st 6 thoracic vertebrae	mastoid and occiput	extends, hyperextends head, neck; acting on one side, they laterally flex, rotate head, neck

Index